Somethin' To Shout About!

By
Donna Green-Goodman, MPH

SOMETHIN' TO SHOUT ABOUT!!

Celebrating Health and Healing Through Diet and Lifestyle

Includes Delicious Vegan/Vegetarian Recipes

By

Donna Green-Goodman, M.P.H.

foreword by

David L. Moore, M.D.

SOMETHIN' TO SHOUT ABOUT!!

Celebrating Health and Healing Through Diet and Lifestyle

Donna Green-Goodman, M.P.H.

Table of Contents

and Marv, and their families, for celebrating with me in my anointing service.

Aunt Jeannie and Uncle Marshall and Dr. & Mrs. Samuel DeShay, for encouraging me to "stay faithful".

Cynthia "Cindy" Allen - my college classmate and God-sent secret sister.

Staff at the Office of Nutrition, GA Division of Public Health.

Thomas Westbrook Goggin, MD, ob/gyn, for respecting the role of lifestyle in his treatment of me.

Staff at Wildwood Lifestyle Center and Hospital, Scott Grivas, MD, Annie and Mary.

Decatur SDA Church family, for prayers and food - especially Thelma Peterson, Julia Miller, Mattie Donwell and Stephanie Seay.

Desiree Goodman, my mother-in-law, for her example of being anointed for a terminal disease, many years ago. You're still here!

Pat Drummond, my sister-in-law, for her frankness about my recipes when I first started developing them.

Carmen Hunt, my niece, for being willing to try a new lifestyle, with great success.

My Loma Linda University SPH professors - Joyce Hopp, The Registers, Richard Neil, Ella Haddad, Albert Sanchez, Winston Craig, and Patricia Johnston, for documenting through research this wonderful lifestyle, and training thousands of students to spread the word.

The Lifestyle Principles, Inc., family.

Debbie, Judy, and Mommy, for helping out with the Lifestyle for Better Health Seminars.

All the **people** who attend the **Lifestyle For Better Health Seminars.**

Pam, Pat and Greg at the **ABC Christian Bookstore** in Decatur, GA

Black Vegetarian Society of Georgia

Connie Flint, Esmond Patterson, Franz Lynch and the 1380
WAOK family.

Victoria Joiner- Miller and the staff at WOCG-FM, 90.1, the Light
of the Tennessee Valley.

Edrene Malcolm, Judith McCoy and Aunt Frances Bliss, *living*
witnesses to what God can do with Breast Cancer.

Regina Barnes and Pamela Byoune - when I grow up!!

India Medley - who has been a prayer warrior friend for many years.

Kristen Betts, Edna Brown, Sonia Paul, Leon Seard, MD, Phyllis
Watkins, and Linda Webb true examples of love and support.

Aunt Marie and Uncle Melvin, for your prayers and calls.

Jennifer Bent - your belief in my vision. Touch and agree, believe and
receive!!

My neighbor Frank Johnson and the pastoral staff and members of
Stronghold Christian Church for their prayers.

Annie Carr, Vera Green, Donna Henry, registered dietitians who
really believe in the power of a plant-based diet.

Leonard Jack, Jr., Ph.D., a man who honors God in his body temple.

Hundreds of Oakwood College students who passed through our
home or restaurant "Chub's", inspiring us to develop delicious,
nutritious dishes.

Many, many other family, loved ones and friends who have
encouraged me and my family.

Laura Hunter-Valcin, Terry Moreland and Tarry Nwaise, without
whom this book could never have been.

9

I am certain you will be blessed as you read this book and will want to obtain copies for friends and loved ones who may be struggling with physical maladies, or for those who need to eat more healthfully.

May God's blessing be with you as you read this inspirational and educational book.

David L. Moore, M.D.

MY STORY

JOURNEY TO HEALING

Journey to Healing

I believe that I was created by a loving God who placed me on this earth to do something in a way that only I could. Many times we focus on the doing, and we tend to want to bypass the journey we must take to really become the person we were created to be. Sometimes, it's painful. I surely wasn't expecting breast cancer. That's one of those diseases that strikes terror in your heart. Today, however, I can't imagine my life without it. It's been a daily act of faith. But, my faith has been strengthened by exercise. Wherever you are in your life, whatever you may be facing, realize that you are being tenderly cared for, and you will come out shoutin'.

The following promises have helped to make my journey to healing, not just from cancer, but from so much other stuff, able to bear. May you be blessed by them and the story of my experience.

"Beloved, think it not strange concerning the fiery trial which is to try you, as though some strange thing happened unto you: but rejoice,...that, when His glory shall be revealed, ye may be glad also with exceeding joy." 1 Peter 4: 12, 13

"In the full light of day, and in hearing of the music of other voices, the caged bird will not sing the song that his master seeks to teach him. He learns a snatch of this, a trill of that, but never a separate and entire melody. But the master covers the cage and places it where the bird will listen to the one song he is to sing. In the dark, he tries and tries again to sing that song until it is learned, and he breaks forth in perfect melody. Then the bird is brought forth, and ever after he can sing that song in the light. Thus God deals with his children. He has a song to teach us, and when we have learned it amid the shadows of affliction, we can sing it ever afterward.

Ellen G. White, Ministry Of Healing, p. 472

"I will not die but live, and proclaim what the Lord has done. The Lord has chastened me severely, but He has not given me over unto death." Psalm 117:18, 19

Before the world was formed, God had you on His mind
He knew the joys and pain you'd face and hoped that
you would find,
He allows these things to happen, For he knows the
plans He has for you;
And He has promised in His Word that He will bring
you through.
He will bring you through, He has something only you
can do
Hold fast to His promises, You will come forth as pure
gold!
And when He brings you out,
He'll give you "Somethin' to Shout About!"
Trust my Jesus, He knows what's best for you.

Donna Green-Goodman
5/99

Diagnosis! Breast Cancer!!

In May of 1996, I was about to get a major wake-up call and my life would be changed forever. I had just returned from five wonderful PHYSICIAN RECOMMENDED days in Nassau, Bahamas with my husband. During my annual visit to my ob/gyn, he could tell when examining me that there was no physical reason for the symptoms of which I complained - tiredness, inability to sleep, etc. He could also tell, by looking at my skin, which he said is the largest organ of my body, that something was not right. He figured that since I was a full-time professional woman, as well as a full-time wife and mother, giving everyone 100% of myself, I had probably overextended myself and perhaps was a little depressed. Upon questioning my husband and me, he discovered that we could not even remember the last time we had gone away ALONE together for an extended vacation. He told us to make reservations immediately for CANCUN, (a place where he had taken his office staff to refuel) or a reasonable facsimile. And, we were to let him know as soon as the reservations were made. We found a reasonably priced trip to Nassau, made the reservations, arranged to fly through Miami, where we would drop off our seven year old son with his grandparents, packed the island stuff and headed for the airport.

Upon arrival in the Bahamas, it was raining, but already I could sense the calming influence of another place--a place where no one would be asking me to pass them this, fix them that, complete a report etc, etc. This was JUST what the doctor ordered. I used those five days strictly to **R-E-L-A-X**. NOTHING, not even the gentle insistence of my husband could move me from the beach lounge chair where I soaked up sun-rays (yes, it did stop raining) and drank any type of virgin fruit drink I could get my hands on. I read, I slept, I laughed, I cried, I expressed my love to my husband, I prayed...I prayed a lot. My final treat to myself was at one of the hotel spas, where after an aerobic workout, I enjoyed a full body massage complete with use of jacuzzi, sauna, and steamroom. When I finally left the spa, I wandered-quite relaxed-through the hotel lobby in and out of gift shops. So relaxed was I that I did not even sense my husband watching me from the hallway ... as I was spending money! What a way to shop!! When our plane lifted off to come home, I CRIED! This was one feeling that I did not want to soon let go. I was definitely going to have to make some changes in my life upon return to the mainland.

Now, while I was in the Bahamas, I knew that I'd had a mammogram before we left home. About ten years before, I'd had a fibroadenoma removed without any complications. Another lump had grown in the same breast location that looked like, felt like, and acted like the previous one. My ob/gyn and I followed it carefully watching for any change. This year, however, we decided to do a mammogram "just to be sure". But I knew that everything would be just fine when I returned. Little did I know that our lives were about to take a major detour because of what was discovered by the physicians. Upon return, I spoke with my physician, thanking him for insisting that we go and describing the wonderful time we'd had while away. He was happy for us, but shared with me that the mammogram had indicated some calcifications that might be suspicious. I needed to have another mammogram done in order to look more closely at what they saw. He assured me that the odds were in my favor and this was just to be sure. I got the second mammogram. Because the radiation technician took so many pictures, I started to wonder if something was wrong. But, I really could not let it pre-occupy my time because I was about to fly to Portland, Oregon to make a presentation at a national meeting. Since my husband and I had left our son in Florida for a few weeks, both of us were going to be able to go to Portland and mix a little pleasure with business.

We went and had a wonderful time. Beach, mountains, waterfront fair, late nights and later mornings. We even got to see some family that my husband had never met. Two vacations in a month. I am really on a roll now.

Upon return from the Portland trip, I was called by my physician. He told me that the calcifications were indeed suspicious, and I needed to see a surgeon for a consultation. I should speak with his office manager to get the name of the surgeon and set up an appointment for the consultation. I was sitting at my desk at work when I got the call. All of a sudden, I was hot all over and everything that was going on around me became a blur. Two of my sister colleagues that I would have spoken with had already left for the day...so all I could do was pack up my stuff and head for the elevator. Someone is asking me something, I really can't process what they are saying. God, just get me to my car. Driving home was a blur...amid the tears that were flowing were the thoughts of cancer and death ... MY God what are you trying to teach me?! I am trying to get my life in balance. Why is this happening now? This is not happening now. I will get to the surgeon and everything will be alright!!!

When I got home, and was finally able to tell my husband what was going on, I was not good! In his ever calm, supportive way, he assured me that we would get through this, whatever the outcome. We prayed together and asked God for direction. I decided that I would go for the consult.

Between that decision and the consult, I was able to talk with my colleague at work. She believed in the importance of balance in life and had a healthy respect for the impact of complementary medicine in one's life. She was so much like me. When I told her what was going on, she suggested that we go to a bookstore at lunch and look for a book on herbal healing for women that she used and was quite impressed with. We went and could not find the book, but spent some wonderful bonding time together. I promised her that I would buy the book and see how it could benefit me. Before I could get my hands on one, she brought me hers, and we discovered some specific remedies for treating what I **thought** I had.

Of course as all of this is happening, I am re-examining my life. God, if you are telling me anything at all, it may be that this **superwoman stuff** is *not* what life is really about. Maybe it is time for me to get back fully in touch with You and what Your plan for my life is. I decided to cancel my next conference (scheduled for a beach location) and take some time off to think, pray and address the health issues I was facing.

As I was leaving the office one day to go to see the doctor, I bumped into one of my colleagues who did not know what was going on. When I explained it to her, she starts crying, hugs me and all of a sudden, I am comforting her and saying, "Cathy, it's going to be alright. God has allowed this and He will se me through it."

When I got to the surgeon's office he said, "These calcifications are suspicious in appearance. We can take one of two approaches: 1. We can biopsy it immediately, or 2. We can watch it for three months to see if there are any changes and then biopsy it." I told him I would make a decision after I talked with my husband about it, and I left the office.

In this age of medicine, not to get a second opinion is to commit self-destruction. Since this surgeon was actually in another city, I decided to look for someone locally. I immediately went in search of a physician in the Atlanta area who could also examine me. I was able to get an appointment with a surgeon and while waiting for the appointed time, I spent about 10 days doing nothing more stressful than reading, sun-bathing, applying herbal treatments, drinking herbal tea, listening to CeCe Winans *Alone in His Presence* tape and praying. I also spoke by phone with Wildwood Lifestyle Center and Hospital, a preventive medicine hospital whose recommendation to me was to immediately **stop eating any and all animal products,** processed foods, start juicing carrots and beets and get plenty of sun and rest. I did exactly as they told me. The lady on the end of the phone line ended our conversation with prayer. She asked God to make known His presence to me as I faced the unknown. She assured me that **He** is the Great Physician and knows what is best for me. He was holding me in the palm of His hand as He knew before I was even conceived that this day would come.

When the day finally arrived to go to the doctor for the second opinion, my husband and I went together. We gave her my history, she examined me and wisely suggested an **immediate** biopsy. It seems that the next few weeks were a BIG BLUR. I went in for out-patient surgery, was biopsied and was told that they removed a big mass and would not be able to confirm anything until the pathology report was returned. I did a lot of praying, and crying, and questioning as I waited to hear from her. I rationalized that okay, I just knew it was going to be benign, or in the early stage. You eat right, exercise and do breast self-examinations. Not to worry. Five days later, with my husband and my little sister/friend, Cynthia Brame by my side, I was told that I did indeed have infiltrating ductal carcinoma. I would need additional surgery to determine how extensive it was and what treatment to take.

Okay, Jesus, I need to feel your presence. My parents are en route here and this is not what any of us were expecting. What should I do?? We made the necessary arrangements for the next surgery and waited to see what was going to happen.

In between surgeries I spoke with my friends from all over the country. Some of them were medical professionals and were quite helpful to my husband and me. One friend, Dr. Leon Seard re-explained what the doctors had said but in a calm, clear, understandable way.

After the next surgery, which was more invasive, my husband and I went for the follow-up visit. The surgeon removed my drain, examined the incision site, and dropped the bomb--- the cancer had already metastasized and was in 6 of 17 lymph nodes that had been removed, the cancer cells themselves were a very

21

aggressive form, and because of my age and race I was at serious risk for death within 2-5 years. I was stunned.

She wanted me to start the most aggressive treatment there was for women like me which would include radiation and massive doses of chemotherapy. She immediately scheduled me for a bone scan, chest x-ray and cat scan of my liver. She gave me the names of two oncologists to visit as well as a radiation therapist. She also wanted me to consider having a stem cell transplant which would cost at least $100,000.00, and it was not covered by insurance! I was assured that once the process was begun, a source of funding for my procedure would be found. She probably said a lot more, but I didn't hear it.

When we went to the front desk, the receptionist, with whom I was developing a real rapport, could tell that I was in shock. "Girl, pull it together. You will get through this. You have God and a wonderful husband who is with you every time you come in here. A lot of women get dropped by their men as soon as they are diagnosed." I thanked her and left. When we got to the car, my husband confessed that he had been told immediately after the first surgery that it was cancer. The doctor had not wanted me to worry. For nearly a month, he had carried that information, all while being attentive to and supportive of me.

My husband and I never stopped praying and after one consult with our friend Dr. Leon Seard, we pretty much decided that I would go to the preventive medicine hospital in Wildwood, Georgia for a visit and come back and do the radiation and chemotherapy. But that was before all my visits to the specialists.

Over the next few weeks, I visited all of the doctors my surgeon wanted me to see. I had what seemed like a gazillion more pictures taken of more parts of my body than I knew I had. The more I spoke to them and read their information, the less impressed I was with their recommendations to me. During none of the visits did anyone stop to even ask me if anything else was going on in my life. No one cared that within the space of three years:

- ♦ I was having major marital problems.
- ♦ My father was diagnosed with colon cancer, and we began regular treks to Florida.
- ♦ One of my students at the school at which I taught was killed in a Freaknik weekend car accident.
- ♦ My husband lost his job.
- ♦ We lost our health insurance.
- ♦ I changed jobs.
- ♦ We moved to another city so my son could attend a private, Christian school.
- ♦ We had put our house on the market and were paying two notes for a while.
- ♦ We kept two growing, hungry teenagers in our home free of charge so they could attend the same Christian school our son attended.
- ♦ Another one of my students was in the last stages of AIDS and died.
- ♦ I had been experiencing a number of female problems and I had to have surgery.
- ♦ We moved back to Georgia.

- ♦ We both started new jobs and new lives. My son started a new school.
- ♦ My Aunt Priss was diagnosed with inoperable cancer.
- ♦ I was stuck in a job that was stressful.
- ♦ My father's cancer recurred.
- ♦ During my father's convalescence, my brother arrived (I think for back-up) and announced that he has AIDS. His T-cells were so low and health so poor that his friends gave him a birthday party a month before his birthday because it was doubtful that he would live to see another birthday.
- ♦ I am stressed to the max and not taking care of myself like I should.

And, now the doctor's diagnose me with aggressive breast cancer and have the **nerve** to tell me that because I was **black and 37**, I could really do nothing other than what they said with any type of positive outcome. Like I chose to be born when I was and be the color I am---"Well, those little details are God's problem," I thought. He said "Before I formed thee in the belly I knew thee..." Jeremiah 1:4, 5. When I explained to one oncologist that I believed in God, he quickly said that he did too, but that wasn't enough. I had to have this chemo or else I would die. Another oncologist, who had great bedside manner, did acknowledge after reviewing my chart and examining me, that she didn't know much about people who practiced healthful lifestyles and their cancer risk and/or survival. She just hoped I wasn't a Jehovah's Witness because I would need lots of blood transfusions, and she knew they didn't do that. She told me that 65-70% of the women with my type of cancer did not survive. When I asked her what happened to the other 25-30%, she said she didn't know. No one was following them. I was given the name and number of a special research project that was going on at Emory University and was encouraged to call them. Maybe if I fit the protocol, I could be added to their study. The lady I spoke with meant well. She just could not understand, how I could refuse a standard treatment that would not guarantee my life but would cause hair loss, bone marrow depression, digestive tract problems, and early menopause, among other things. She flat out told me that she could guarantee my death in 2-5 years without standard treatment, since my cancer was so aggressive.

SOMETHING IS WRONG WITH THIS PICTURE. People who know nothing about me, and don't seem to want to know much beyond what I clinically present, expect me to let them take over my life with an experimental procedure that offers no guarantees. By the end of that conversation, she was positive that I had a faith in God so that no matter the outcome, I was gonna be alright.

At my next visit to the surgeon, I was supposed to be able to lift my arm overhead. I could not. My husband, who is a physical therapist, promised that in three days I would be able to do it. We left the office en route to a CeCe Winans concert. My secret sister had sent me tickets earlier as a gift. Never in my life had a gospel concert meant so much to me. CeCe ministered to my soul! In between sets of songs, and meeting the people and testifying, my husband gave me stretching exercises. By the time the concert was over you know where both my arms were! Umm huh! Up in the air. Glory, Hallelujah.

Encounter With the Enemy!

I had been talking it over with Jesus since the first surgery, and I was becoming convinced more and more that I needed a physician who was genuinely guided by the Great Physician. I knew what I must do.

When I went for my next visit to the doctor, she tried her best to get me to do things her way. I told her what I planned to do. She suggested I talk it over with my husband because he might feel differently. I told her that he agreed wholeheartedly with me. She, of course, was not happy. She told me that I was taking a risk she would not recommend, but she realized that we were not to be dissuaded.

After a phone consult with Dr. Scott Grivas, a Preventive Lifestyle physician, I made the final decision to go to Wildwood Lifestyle Center and Hospital in Wildwood, Georgia for their ten-day treatment. I made the necessary arrangements and started getting ready for my trip. After making the decision, I received a "peace that passed all understanding". My husband and I sat our child down and explained to him that we had been praying and reading up on Mommy's disease and were convinced that while we could not point to one specific cause for me getting it, there were some things I had done, specifically in the area of our diets that could have contributed to it. I apologized for what I had done, and we told him that I was going to a special hospital for ten days for treatment. They would teach me a new way of life and when I returned, things would be different at home. We said we were going to pray together that Jesus would make the cancer cells so small that they would not be able to multiply and grow in my body and make me sicker. His immediate response was, "No Mommy, we're gonna pray that God makes them disappear so you won't be sick again." The faith of a child! We prayed and believed that God would bless.

After going to bed that night, confident that I had made the right decision, I slept peacefully for several hours. Around 11:00, I was awakened by an intense pressure on my chest. The room was very hot and I was having trouble breathing. I got up and checked my family. They were sound asleep. I moved around quietly, so I wouldn't awaken them. I turned on the attic fan to try to cool the house so I could breathe. I tried to sleep again, but with no success. Then, I felt a strange presence in the room. The pressure on my chest worsened. I started praying and repeating scriptural promises and rehearsing the words to songs of faith that I knew. The pressure on my chest would not give up. I continued to pray and about an hour later, I finally drifted off to sleep. Suddenly, I was awakened by a loud pop! It sounded like it does when lightning strikes something electrical.   I looked outside, and it was pitch black in the subdivision. Okay, it's time for somebody else to wake up!!! I shook my husband awake and relayed what was going on.   We heard our neighbors outside and asked if they knew what had happened. There was not a cloud in the sky, no rain or storms anywhere. But obviously a transformer had blown. We felt for sure that something supernatural was going on. My husband and I began to rehearse what happened, and we realized that something supernatural had just happened. This whole experience I was having was **less** about breast cancer and **more** about the spiritual warfare in which we are engaged. "For we wrestle not against flesh and blood..." Ephesians 6:12. The devil was angry and was trying to kill me. We prayed together and asked God for intervention and protection from the enemy and direction for whatever God had planned for the rest of my life.

The next morning as my husband was leaving for work, the Georgia Power company was repairing the transformer. My husband asked them if they knew what had happened. They could not explain it. There had been no rain or storm in the area the night before, neither had there been any accidents. "Whatever it was had to be mighty powerful to have knocked out the entire subdivision," said the repairman. I knew exactly what had happened. I'd had an encounter with the enemy!

Over the next few days, I was more thoroughly convinced that a spiritual approach to my disease was necessary. I decided part of my treatment would be to have an anointing service, as is outlined in the book of James 5: 14,15 "Is any sick among you: let him call for the elders of the church; and let them pray over him, anointing him with oil in the name of the Lord: And the prayer of faith shall save the sick, and the Lord shall raise him up; and if he have committed sins, they shall be forgiven them."

I contacted our cousin, Elder T. Marshall Kelly to see if he could conduct the service. He could not, but recommended Elder C. Dunbar Henri, Sr., and Elder R .L. Woodfork- two men of God that were long time friends of our family, as well as local ministers. I contacted them, explained my situation and asked if they would anoint me. They agreed. Elder Henri gave me specific counsel. "This is not a service of last rites. We are anointing you to ask God for an intervention. You may have whoever you'd like at the service. Convey to them the seriousness of the service, and ask them not to come if they are not comfortable with the idea or may be practicing something that can **block the blessing**. Confess to others and to God any sins that may be in your life, and we will be at your home at the appointed time." I called a number of my prayer warrior friends and invited them. They were all so happy to attend. I invited friends with children so that my child would not be frightened. We planned a love feast to follow the anointing. I got busy talking to God about things in my life that were not right and made a few calls to people that I needed to... "for if I regard iniquity in my heart, then the Lord will not hear me." Psalm 66:18.

On the appointed Friday evening, right before the Sabbath hours began, my family and friends gathered around sunset for a vesper and anointing service. It was beautiful. There was singing, praying, testifying and the actual anointing service. Many others of my friends around the country knew the time we were gathered and were in prayer as well. The ministers reiterated how serious the service was and that from the day I asked them to officiate, they had begun to pray that they would be worthy vessels for the blessing to flow through. (How different than all of the **physicians** I visited.) They explained that it is **God's power** that can heal us and told us that if it was not His will for me to be healed, that He would see us through it. Both ministers placed their hands on my head and asked God to intervene in my life- if it was His will and could glorify Him. They then put the oil on my forehead and thanked God in advance for whatever He would do, letting Him know that if He spared me, I was under renewed **obligation** to testify of Him, and if it was His will for me to go to sleep, that my soul would be right so that when He returned, I could go to heaven with Him. Needless to say, there was a mighty experience going on in that room that night. When my brother called to see how my mom had made it through, I told him that she didn't have much time to cry, because she was running around handing out tissues to all of my friends. I spoke with my aunt the next day and discovered that she had fallen asleep while waiting for the appointed time to pray. Suddenly, she woke up in a sweat screaming, "Oh, my God, I am supposed to be praying for Donna." When she looked at the clock, it was exactly the time that she was supposed to be praying. Glory, Hallelujah!!

Pathway to a New Lifestyle

O n Monday morning, my husband, father and son drove me to Wildwood Lifestyle Center and Hospital where I would spend the next 10 days. After settling in, I was scheduled to see the doctor. My husband and I and the lifestyle consultant that was assigned to me met the doctor in the examining room. Before putting his hand on me, he asked us to kneel with him in prayer as he sought direction from the Heavenly Physician. His prayer went something like this - "Dear God, I don't know Sister Donna, but You do. You have sent her here to me, and I am asking that You will direct my attention to her so that I will do what You know she needs. And Lord, we will give You all the praise for whatever You do. Thank you for hearing and answering my prayer. Amen" **I KNEW I WAS IN THE RIGHT PLACE.** Following the exam, he wrote out my plan for the next ten days and said we were going to trust God. My family left after lunch and I was on my own. My son Ivey, slipped me a note that read, 'Mommy, I can't wait till you get back and I can taste your new recipes.' The next ten days were an experience I would not soon forget.

Wildwood Lifestyle Center is a Christian medical facility that believes that following simple lifestyle principles is the BEST WAY to health. They believe that God is the true source of healing. And, that by obeying His health laws, we can avoid disease, reduce our risk for disease, and recover health when we experience disease. Patients come to Wildwood for a variety of health problems including heart disease, hypertension, diabetes, obesity, stress, cancer, substance abuse, lupus to name a few. When the patients come to the facility to be admitted or to participate in the Lifestyle Conditioning Programs offered, they are pointed to Christ as the source of **ALL** true healing. Patients are assigned a lifestyle consultant who is a lifeline throughout their stay. The lifestyle consultant provides prescribed treatments as outlined by the admitting physician, participates in presenting the many educational sessions that are offered, and by precept and personal example, offers hope and comfort for the patient's situation. They are such a source of comfort and joy to the many patients dealing with the prospect of death, and struggling to accept how a lifestyle approach to disease has such a dramatic effect on health recovery. I was blessed to have two consultants Mary and Annie.

I was put on the general plan that is prescribed for all patients who come to Wildwood, with additional treatments specific to breast cancer. The diet for all who come to Wildwood is **vegan** (strict vegetarian, absolutely no animal products), which is really what God prescribed for us at the beginning of time. Instead of using toxic chemicals to try to arrest my cancer, I was given daily hydrotherapy treatments and massage which actually work in harmony with the body to stimulate the body's own immune system. Since hormone imbalance was part of my problem, I was prescribed several herbal preparations known to help hormonal imbalance. Each day we started with a group morning devotional followed by breakfast and a short walk on one of the many nature trails. After our morning stretching sessions, we would walk again and then participate in lifestyle education seminars, cooking classes and our individualized medical treatment programs. A hearty lunch was served every day followed by another walk and the afternoon was spent learning more about why disease occurs and how we can, through diet and lifestyle, prevent it from occurring. Supper, which was always something very light, was served to the **few** patients on a 3-meal per day plan. After an evening walk, we gathered for one more group session and then retired for the night.

Doctors' rounds proved to be a special blessing. Still frightened by my prognosis the first time Dr. Grivas came to see me all I could say was, "I'm going to die". His calm response was "Sister Donna, you are in the midst of a spiritual warfare. The battle is far bigger than your breast cancer. Satan is trying to kill you, and he doesn't care how he does it. He uses stress, overwork, disease, unhappy relationships and a lot of other things to get us to lose sight of why we are here and where we ultimately want to go...heaven. Some of us **will** die. But, if we do, it will only be for a nap, because the coming of Jesus is so **soon**. And, when he comes, all who have gone to sleep in Him will be called from their dusty graves to life eternal. But, we are not going to even think about death. We are going to ask God to find every cancer cell in your body and get rid of it. *Angels* walk the halls at Wildwood, and we know that it is God who does the healing, not just of your body, but also of your soul."

"At Wildwood" he continued, "we just don't treat

34

symptoms of disease. Whenever we are sick, we must acknowledge it and learn why. Disease never comes without a cause. Most often it happens because we are abusing the laws of health. We must look at the things we are doing and set about correcting the harmful ones and practice those that are more favorable to promoting health. Use only simple methods/treatments that do not harm the body as you work to recover health and realize that the Holy Spirit can renew every organ of the body. When God intervenes in your life and restores your health, you must 'Go and sin no more, lest a worse thing comes unto you.' John 5:14. Then, find out the vision/blueprint God has for you and dedicate the rest of your life to fulfilling it. If you decide to do adjuvant therapy for your breast cancer, do only the minimal, non-invasive type and go only as long as your body can stand it. Trust God to do what is best."

Mary, one of my lifestyle counselors, confirmed his words. "Donna," she said, "when God heals us it can be done in one of three ways. **Instantly**, when He speaks the word; by **simple means**, when He used the clay on the man's eyes, and had Naaman dip in the water; or at the **resurrection,** like what happened to Lazarus."

Well, here I was at a hospital, and it seems like I was at church being lifted up to Jesus. This is feeling real good. Lord, I don't know what your plans are for me, but I am listening and willing to obey.

While at Wildwood, I made new friends, relearned a lot of what I knew, but had not been practicing, and most of all got in touch with Jesus myself. I heard Him talk to me. After the evening walk, I would come back to my room and sit and watch the

35

trees and flowers and just talk to Him. The day I discovered specifically the things I had been doing that could possibly have contributed to my disease, I **ran** to my room and fell on my knees and prayed David's Prayer....Have mercy upon me O God....for I have sinned...I humbly acknowledge my transgressions,...Create in me a clean heart O God and renew a right spirit within me. Psalm 51:1-4,7,10-12. And then I prayed with sincerity of heart,

"Lord, I would never have chosen to have breast cancer. But, You in Your wisdom have allowed it. Since being at Wildwood, I am so encouraged at how You work to heal us and direct us to maintain our health. There are a lot of people I know personally that don't know or cannot afford to come to a place like Wildwood. So Lord, if it is your will to heal me of this devastating disease, please do. And Lord, I **promise** to tell others how they can recover health. I'm gonna need some help Lord. I've heard about this doctor named David Moore who used to work here at Wildwood. If it is your will, could you please work it out so I can work with him in the Atlanta, GA area in a 'ministry of healing'? I thank you Lord for whatever you are going to do. In your name, Amen."

When my husband returned on the 10th day to pick me up, I did not want to leave. This place was too safe and serene and connected to heaven. Lord, what would I face when I got back to the valley? No matter what awaits me, You will be with me. Amidst tears, I piled in the car and headed home. I would do the radiation, maintain my diet and lifestyle changes and leave the rest in God's hands.

The first thing I did when I got home, was to put the trash can to my refrigerator and empty out all the remaining foods that would work against my recovery. My husband and son watched in amazement. Eddie finally blurted out "Are you gonna throw that away too?" "Yes," I replied. "We have asked God to do His part, and now we must do our part as a family to build up our body temples. You do want me to live, don't you?" They agreed and pledged their support. Since I love to cook, I got busy creating delicious foods so they wouldn't even miss what we had surrendered.

Walking By Faith

After settling in at home, I made the arrangements for the radiation and got measured for the treatments. That took a whole morning. I left with instruction to return the next week to begin treatment. The first session would take quite a while because they had to make sure that everything that they had done the first day was correct and that they would be aiming the radiation at the right spot. During the next visit I was marked up, taped up and given instructions not to wash those areas. When the irritation began, I was told to use only aloe vera to relieve the discomfort. The first treatment was so humiliating I cried, right there on the table. The therapist admitted that that was not unusual, and she often went home in tears wondering how women did it. For the next three weeks I went faithfully for my radiation treatment, five days a week. At week four I was so nauseous that I decided that I had to stop. After Friday's treatment, I came home, ran a tub of water and washed all of the marks and tapes off. My body had had enough. I typed and faxed a letter to the physician that stated I was through. My surgeon was again unhappy and tried to convince me to take an oral medication. I declined.

By now it's September and I have missed the Olympics, have a smaller, burned breast and am worn out from radiation treatment. My next doctor's visit is not scheduled until December. I set about maintaining the diet and lifestyle prescribed for me at Wildwood.

At Thanksgiving we celebrate with an old-fashioned

Dinner **vegan** style. My friends Regina, Darleen and Mike join us. We all feel so healthy and happy that we can eat well and it tastes good. I set about sharing my story and recipes with everyone who is interested. God is good! In December, I go for my visit. My blood test results, which were taken in the laboratory, are not in the office when I arrive. I must wait until they arrive to discover the status of my health. A few days later I call and get nothing. Finally, I drop by and one of the office staff members shows me my file which says that my blood levels are elevated. The doctor calls me at home to confirm it and wishes me a happy holiday. **Happy Holiday?** I say!! Well, God, you are in charge. I choose not to even discuss the results with her. It is too close to Christmas; my family deserves a peaceful, stressless, few days. My birthday is coming up in January, I will not even think about what the doctor has said. Whenever I go there it is always worse news.

Then there is this problem with my eye. I can't seem to keep my contact lens in.   After it pops out, and I cannot find it, I go to the eye doctor and discover that with my cancer, the hormone levels have been affected and so has the shape of my eye. She wants to follow up on me because a lot of times when the cancer recurs, it manifests itself in the nerves of the eye.   Oh, Jesus!! It's looking kind of dark right now. The lab report, and now my eye. What is going on? Well, at least those awful PMS symptoms have stopped, my migraines are gone, my skin is clearing up, I'm sleeping better and I don't feel so tired all the time anymore. When I did my breast self examination this month, I could find no fibrocystic lumps, and for the first time in my life, my breasts are as soft as cotton. (My husband concurs). I have lost weight and I can fit those blue jeans I haven't worn since I bought them. I must really walk by faith now and not by sight. I

39

will continue obeying Him no matter what.

In January, I throw myself a birthday party. I invite my friends. The menu is **only** healthy food. They eat it **ALL** up. This is so much fun. When the last guest leaves, I can hardly settle down. I have laughed so much and had so much fun, that I feel like you do when you go roller skating, take off the skates and feel like you are still moving. This is exactly what I needed. "A merry heart really doeth good like a medicine." Proverbs 17:22.

Somethin' To Shout About!!

It's almost April now. Almost time for my next doctor's visit. I am really ready to talk now. I have been so confirmed of God's direction in my life over the last 10 months. Before we go though, we will be attending my college homecoming. (A UNCF school in Alabama) I have so much to be thankful for and so many people to thank for their support. And, you know how the people can be...word on the street is it's all in her lungs...They need to see a miracle! The visit is whirlwind, but very inspiring. We leave there and go to Orlando for a week...just my husband, my son and me. Upon return, I go to the doctor's office. Before going inside, I talk to Jesus. Lord, I trust you. I feel great. I am sometimes weary of the people who don't know You like I do and can only relate to what the blood tests say. Can You please give me some evidence today?

"Hey you two", the surgeon starts the visit. "Whenever you turkeys come to see me" (we're friends now), "I get uneasy because you didn't do what I recommended. Tell me what is going on." I tell her how great I am feeling. She asks if I am experiencing any joint pain...No, I say. How is your diet? Great! After she asks me that the third time I ask her, is something supposed to be wrong? Well, no, I just don't want you losing any weight. I just want to be sure you are eating. My husband confirms that I am most definitely eating well and without any problems!!! She examines me thoroughly and it is noticeable that she seems surprised not to find another lump (even the fibrocystic breast lumps are gone.)   She wants to see me every six months, keep doing what I am doing, not get pregnant and not second guess my decision to approach my disease this way. She says "There are a small number of women who do well with the disease, and she is hoping that I am one. The one thing that traditional practitioners cannot put their hands on and quantify is the body's immune system. A person's immune system is what determines how well a person actually does. Some women with poor prognoses do well, and some with good prognoses don't do well. So just keep doing what you're doing."

We ask for an explanation of the December test results. The ones that were supposed to be elevated. She explains that there was absolutely no indication of metastasis in the lung area. The blood tests show all levels in the normal range:

Breast Cancer Tumor Markers **CA 27-29**- Normal range is 0-37

Mine started at 22 and dropped to 15 then to 12

General Cancer Tumor Marker **CEA**-Normal Range is 0-5

Mine is at less than .5

I ask if that means that I am in remission. She explains no, not really. If I had followed her recommendation and gotten this result, they would call this a cure; if the disease recurs, they would treat it again and then I would be in remission. My husband asks her, so what do you call this?   Stammer, stutter........"I guess we would call this a cure," she says. My head nearly explodes. My eyes catch those of my husbands and we have **"Somethin' to Shout About!"** But since we are in the doctor's office we are both **shouting** silently...Glory, Hallelujah!! He **IS** able to KEEP YOU FROM FALLING!!!! Jude 24.   When she leaves the examination room, we embrace and thank God immediately.   This did not just happen, the blessing was granted in August, I am just realizing it. "Before you call , I will answer....while you are yet speaking, I will hear." Isaiah 65:24. "For I am the Lord that Healeth thee...who forgiveth all thine iniquities, who healeth all thy diseases." Exodus 15:26; Psalms 103:3

Now it's starting to make sense. God intervened in my life in August. My breast cancer was hormone dependent, and as I adopted a lifestyle, including strict dietary habits, I had stopped "feeding" my health problems. As my hormones normalized, my tummy size reduced. The abdominal swelling caused by my uterine fibroids/polyps, my PMS weight gain, breast tenderness, fibrocystic breast disease, irritability, mood swings, migraine headaches, skin eruptions, constipation, cracked and dried lips, leg and back cramps were ALL gone. My periods had changed to two wonderful pain-free days. All my between period spotting had disappeared. My weight had normalized. I was sleeping better. My singing voice had dropped from 2nd soprano back to the alto range I sang in high school. I was responding much better to stress (my daddy was dying). The muscle spasms that used to make my back feel like a brick were gone. The change I experienced in December with my eye, must have been related to the hormones, as the optometrist had said, except that my eyesight was improving.

My husband, who had suffered with heal spurs, no longer had them. My son, who had suffered with seasonal allergies since he was a baby, was allergy free. Our entire family was experiencing an increase in the number of bowel movements we were having. And they weren't smelly anymore! And sex! Don't get me started! We are fearfully and wonderfully made. Obedience to God's plan for health had wrought miracles in our home that the doctors didn't even know about.

I race to the car phone and call my best friend Joann Dickson-Smith. I tell her what just happened in the office. "Did she say healed Donna?" "No", I responded. "Donna, they can't say healed because that's out of their realm. They don't quite understand that this is all spiritual Donna, and they can't heal. **ONLY GOD** can do that!!!!" I spent the next few days calling any and everyone that has been involved in this situation **shoutin'** about the MIRACLE I am experiencing. There are a few who are guarded in their happiness for me. After all, this is not happening according to medical protocol. It could return, you know. I don't want you to be too excited and then be let down. But you know what, I cannot **EVEN** go there with them... Because **I KNOW** the man from Galilee. I have just touched the hem of His garment. And right now, this healing seems really big, but when I stop to think about it, it is only one in a series of blessings. And it is those blessings that have enabled me to trust Him totally with this experience. You see, when I think about all the good things that He has done for me, I just can't tell it all. I know that He has already been with me and helped me to rise above my problems. I remember when

*My car blew up and I wasn't in it.

*Healed my marriage (that man has not always been the wonderful man he is today).

*He led us to our house with the exact amount of money we needed to close.

*The hospital bill was due, check in the mail, I wouldn't open it cause I thought it was another bill.

*He turn my brother's AIDS around.

*He reversed my father's cancer.

*He gave my husband Eddie a promotion when I had to stop working.

*He strengthened me to be able to work some when Eddie was demoted.

*He sent my son's tuition money when we needed it.

*He wouldn't let us get carpet until the water pipes burst, so we wouldn't lose our money.

*He keeps my family safe on the highway--EVERYDAY.

*He daily talks with me and directs me.

He leads me above each and every trap the devil sets for me, if **I am willing to listen to Him and follow his promptings.** His promptings are our enablings. And, he does the same thing for you. He woke you up this morning. You are alive and reading this book....for a reason. Your life may not be exactly what you want it to be, but then what can you really be if you are not what He has planned for you to be? When we stop complaining and start counting blessings, we find out just how good God is. I have learned from this experience, **IF IT IS NOT TERMINAL, YOU CAN HANDLE IT.** Whatever you are going through, you can rise above it, you can have JOY, you can be a partner with Him and you can be a witness to others. You can point those around you to the Savior who gives you the HEALING!! You too can have **Somethin' to Shout About!!!!**

Lifestyle Principles,
Your BEST WAY to Health!

When I asked God to heal me, I also asked for the opportunity to share my story through a medical ministry. I specifically asked that I have the chance to work with Dr. David Moore. Dr. Moore was a Christian physician that my daddy had told me about. He had, at one time, been on staff at Wildwood Lifestyle Center and Hospital in Wildwood, Georgia (the place where I went). And he had been medical director at another lifestyle center in New York called Living Springs Retreat. I figured that if God would allow it, I could work with him and a staff of other qualified people in lifestyle medicine and make a difference in the health of people in the Atlanta, Georgia area. The only barrier to that happening was that he and his family lived in Charlotte, NC. Little did I know that this was all a part of God's plan. In February 1998, God moved Dr. Moore and his family to Atlanta. God led a nurse to us, Jill Kennedy, who was trained as a Lifestyle Counselor and shared our desire for medical ministry.

For months, a group of us met regularly to pray and ask for God's direction for medical ministry in the Atlanta area. On Thursday, November 5, 1998, we celebrated the grand opening of **Lifestyle Principles, Inc., in Decatur, Georgia.** a non-profit corporation founded for the promotion of better physical, mental and spiritual health. Its members firmly believe that *Lifestyle* **is the BEST WAY** to reach optimal health. The corporation offers a multifaceted community health promotion approach to health in the metro-Atlanta area. People can attend health education seminars, hear the latest on preventive lifestyle health via radio, access preventive lifestyle health care at the physician's office, read the office newsletter, support their new way of life when dining out and shopping for good health. Patients are supported and encouraged by a sensitive, caring and spiritual staff, many of whom have recovered health through the principles promoted by Lifestyle Principles, Inc.

LPI's staff includes Dr. Moore, who was trained in traditional medicine at Meharry Medical College. Pam Moore is the receptionist and Dr. Moore's wife. Jill Kennedy-Hutchinson is the nurse and provides hydrotherapy for the female patients and Eddie Goodman, a physical therapist, (and my husband) treats the male hydrotherapy patients. I am the health educator and share my testimony and practical ways of living with the patients. The plant-based recipes in this book are ones I developed or modified to keep my family and friends **enjoying** eating healthy, familiar foods.

Dr. Moore is heard weekly on "Principles for Better Health", a live call-in show on Atlanta's **Gospel** Choice, 1380 WAOK. He is also heard weekly on Oakwood College radio station (Huntsville, Alabama), 90.1 FM - WOCG-The **Light** of the Tennessee Valley, which is accessible via computer. Many others of our group have skills that have helped this dream become a reality, and will continue to help to develop it to God's full potential for it. We are expecting God to provide the means to maintain the office and to establish and maintain a lifestyle conditioning program, as well as a health food store and restaurant.

Our medical approach is scientifically sound, safe, sensible, and scriptural. We work in partnership with the Great

47

Physician.   Our staff models the lifestyle principles that we recommend to patients. And, we don't just tell you what you need to do, we show you how to do it.

LPI is witnessing amazing results in patients/participants health who begin to adopt new lifestyle habits.   Increased consumption of a plant-based diet with reduction in fat consumption, a primary **lifestyle** habit that LPI promotes, has resulted in **major** improvement in the health of patients/participants suffering from or at risk for a range of chronic lifestyle diseases including cancer, heart disease, and diabetes.   Among the patient population, dependence on prescribed medication is reduced, blood circulation has improved (neuropathy), blood levels for cancer tumor markers, cholesterol, triglycerides dropped, blood pressure and glucose levels normalized.   Listed below are documented examples of LPI observed improved patient outcomes after adopting a plant-based diet as a primary lifestyle habit:

> **Mid fifties African-American male** in chemotherapy treatment for lung cancer. Patient unable to complete full round, because of drop in white blood cell count. After adopting a plant-based diet as a main component of lifestyle treatment, patient completed course of chemotherapy without any drop in white blood cell count.

> **32 year old   African-American**   female diagnosed with leiomyosarcoma. CT scan and liver biopsy showed liver metastasis, CT scan showed lung metastasis. Patient refused chemotherapy and adopted a plant-based diet as primary component of lifestyle treatment. Patient indicated 3 lb. weight loss and CT scan negative except liver mass present but reduced in size at follow-up scan.

> **51 year old African-American** female 20 year history of Type 2 Diabetes with neuropathy, hypertension, hypothyroidism, elevated cholesterol, cardiomyopathy, joint swelling, asthma, on **14** prescribed medications to **control symptoms**. Patient followed physician advice, adopting plant-based dietary as primary lifestyle change.

Four months later on medication reduced to 4, has lost 53 lbs., fasting blood sugar dropped from 192 to 115, neuropathy symptoms improved, blood pressure changed from 136/80 to 124/86, patient more self-confident.

48 year old African-American male with a 13 year history of Type 2 Diabetes. On glucophage 2 times per day. Patient adopted plant-based dietary, reduced glucophage to 1 time per day and experienced the following results:	
3/16/99 blood chemistry profile	6/21/99 blood chemistry profile
Glucose - 186	Glucose - 98
Cholesterol - 237	Cholesterol - 204
Triglycerides - 373	Triglycerides - 113
Chol/HDL - 5.2	Chol/HDL - 2.3
HDL - 46	HDL - 89
LDL - 116	LDL - 92

With so much disease and disability in this country related to lifestyle habits, everybody knows somebody who is looking for something to improve their health. At Lifestyle Principles Inc., we believe that health is a gift from God. Because He is equal opportunity, it's hard to imagine Him having you pay for a product that you are on typically, for the rest of your life that really only treats symptoms. That means only people with money could get well. We believe that there are **Lifestyle Principles** that are really your **BEST WAY** to Health! Whatever your lot in life: rich, poor, black, white, educated, uneducated, young or old, if you begin to practice these principles, you can significantly reduce your risk for many diseases, improve your current disease state and

49

recover your health.

Take a close look at the following **Lifestyle Principles**. As you begin to adopt them into your daily life, I guarantee, you will have better health. **Lifestyle Principles, your BEST WAY to Health**!

B - Bedtime Regularity

E - Exercise

S - Sunshine & Simple Diet

T - Temperance

W - Water

A - Air

Y - Yielding to Divine Power

BEDTIME REGULARITY

"Come unto me all ye that labor and are heavy laden and I will give you rest." Matthew 11:28

> *With all that was going on in my life, bedtime was anything but regular. When I went to bed, I would lay there for hours listening to the clock beep every thirty minutes. Sleep was not restful, and I was always tired when I woke up. At Wildwood, I ran to bed at 9:30 p.m. and was so refreshed in the morning. How important is sleep and rest?*

During sleep, the body is repaired. All its activities lessen - less heat is produced, the breathing is slower, the heart beats more slowly, digestion is lessened, the nerves and muscles are relaxed. The entire system is slowed down, and the body building cells carry on their recuperative work.

To receive the greatest benefit from sleep, consider the following:

1. Have regular hours for sleep. By sleeping at regular hours every night, the health, spirits, memory, and the attitude are improved. Irregular hours of sleeping cause the brain forces to be sapped.

2. Have an abundant supply of fresh air during sleep. Sore throats, lung diseases and liver disorders occur when there is not a continuous supply of fresh air during sleep. Also, one wakes up feeling exhausted and feverish from the lack of oxygen. But, when there is a supply of fresh air while sleeping, a sound sweet sleep is

induced.

3. The stomach should have its work all done that it may rest as well as the other organs while sleeping. When the stomach is not empty before sleep, the digestive process continues during the sleeping hours and this results in unpleasant dreams. Since the stomach has worked while you were sleeping, you awaken unrefreshed in the morning and with little desire for a hearty breakfast. You may also experience the feeling of an unsettled stomach and/or nausea.

4. Early to bed and early to rise. The greatest amount of restoration is done to the body during deep sleep. Studies show that, due to the "circadian rhythm: which is regulated by the sun's rays, the deepest sleep occurs between 9 p.m. and 12 midnight.

5. Persons who rest on the 7th day experience a joy unbeknownst to those who don't.

6. Persons who plan recreational vacations are rejuvenating their lives.

When you can't sleep
1. Take a warm bath.
2. Have a cup of chamomile, catnip, skullcap, hops or lady's slipper tea.
3. Listen to some soothing music.
4. Turn **off** the craziness on TV and do some spiritual reading instead.
5. Count your blessings as part of your end of day conversation with God.

EXERCISE

"In the name of Jesus Christ of Nazareth rise up and *WALK!*"
Acts 3:6

> *I prided myself that I worked out 2-3 times per week at a local woman's spa. Little did I realize that the constant pounding and muscle exertion I endured was more than my body needed and could actually have done more harm than good. Simple walking and useful labor afford the necessary benefit of exercise to the body without the possibility of harmful injury. While at Wildwood, every day after every meal and any other time we liked, we took walks through the trails in the fresh air.*

Here's what happens when you *exercise:*

1. It increases circulation.
2. The heart rate increases to pump necessary oxygen to each muscle.
3. It increases the stroke volume, the amount of blood pumped with each heart beat.
4. It decreases the pulse rate, thereby giving the heart more time to rest between beats.
5. It decreases one's risk of death in the event of a heart attack.
6. The lungs are expanded and thus strengthened to supply fresh oxygen to the entire system.
7. Liver, kidneys, and lungs will be strengthened to perform their work.
8. Exercise invigorates the mind.
9. Digestion is aided, a diseased stomach is relieved, and the

bowels are strengthened for correct elimination.

10. Impurities are expelled from the system.

11. The skin expels impurities that otherwise would have to be expelled by the excretory organs, and the skin is given a healthy glow.

12. It increases weight loss.

13. You sleep better.

14. You are less affected by stress.

SUNSHINE

"But unto you that fear my name shall the SUN of righteousness arise with healing in His wings. Malachi 4:2

> *I went to graduate school in California. Our dormitory roof was always full of women after a little more color. Since I was born with plenty of melatonin, they often wondered why I was on the roof. The sunlight has always been such an energizer to me. I knew how it gave our bodies Vitamin D. I learned it also has lots of other benefits when not overused.*

Here's what moderate exposure to **SUNSHINE** can do for you!

1. It helps convert a cholesterol-like substance in our bodies to Vitamin D.

2. It increases the circulation and enables the red blood cells to carry more oxygen.

3. It imparts a healthy tone to the mind and nervous system.

4. It prevents and counteracts mental depression (SAD-Seasonal Affective Disorder)

5. It increases the number of white blood cells in the body.

6. It stimulates the liver to properly perform its functions.

7. It stimulates body functions through the pineal gland, which in turn benefits the pituitary gland which controls the hormone production of other endocrine glands including the liver, pancreas, thyroid and adrenal glands.

8. It lowers the level of blood sugar in the blood stream when it is too high and raises the level if it is too low.

9. When you combine sunbathing with a regular program of exercise, fatigue and exhaustion tend to be reduced and the ability for work is increased. This is due to an increase of glycogen content in the blood and muscles following exercise in the sunlight. The pulse rate is lowered, because the heart muscle is pumping more blood at each beat. This enables your heart to rest more between beats. And yet, the blood output is increased by an average of 39% for several days after a sunbath.

10. A high level of triglycerides, the amount of fats in the blood and a high blood pressure are both lowered by adequate sunlight. Simply taking sunlight on the body will lower the blood pressure. And, when a person combines exercise with receiving sunlight, high blood pressure is lowered even more.

11. Sunlight is known to kill certain germs on exposure. It also promotes the healing of wounds.

SIMPLE DIET

"Behold I have given you every herb yielding seed...And every tree in which is the fruit of a tree yielding seed; to you it shall be for meat." Genesis 1:29

> *Having been a lacto-ovo vegetarian all my life, I pretty much figured I was doing all I could to reduce my risk for disease. After my diagnosis, I reviewed a lot of other information that I already knew and realized that I needed to do more. French fries, chocolate, cheese, ice cream, soft drinks, eating more than I really needed to, had to GO!!! It was time for me to be a vegan! Subsisting wholly on fruits, nuts, grains and vegetables in as unrefined a state as possible would be my new way of life. God has placed amazing SECRETS in the plant world.*

The American Dietetic Association, in its position paper on Vegetarian Diet (Journal of ADA, November 1997, Volume 97, Number) 11 states that "Appropriately planned vegetarian diets are healthful, are nutritionally adequate, and provide health benefits in the prevention and treatment of certain diseases."

Adam and Eve lived in a garden. They subsisted on fruits, nuts, and grains. When they left the garden, vegetables were added. Scientists are discovering that those very foods are loaded, not only with the vitamins and nutrients we are familiar with, but they include a substance called fiber that is **ONLY** found in plant foods. And they are now naming other substances called phytochemicals **ONLY** found in plant foods whose primary *known* function is to enable the body to resist disease. The chronic lifestyle diseases that so many people are suffering and dying from

57

today are especially benefitted. Samuel L. DeShay, MD, a physician in the Maryland/Washington, DC area, was a missionary to Africa for some 12 years. He and his wife Bernice, a registered nurse, cared for this population, who subsists primarily on plant foods. During their tenure there, **not** ONE of the native patients they saw had heart disease. The one case of heart disease that they **did** see was in a missionary of European descent. A plant based diet:

1. Is nutritionally sound.
2. Is economical
3. Disease preventing/health promoting
4. Increases energy
5. Improves overall physical appearance
6. Increases permanent weight loss
7. Improves gastrointestinal function
8. Reduces levels of serum cholesterol and triglycerides
8. Reduces blood pressure in those with hypertension
9. Reduces risk of death from heart disease
10. Reduces risk of kidney/gall bladder disease
11. Reduces insulin requirements
12. Reduces risk of ALL **cancers**
13. Reduces female disorders
14. Reduces **ARTHRITIS** pain
15. Improves sexual function
16. Reduces desire for stimulants like alcohol and tobacco and other drugs
17. Was God's original plan - Genesis 1:29
18. Is what is on heaven's menu - Revelation 21:4, 22:2

TEMPERANCE

"And every man that striveth for the mastery is temperate in all things." 1 Corinthians 9:25

When the doctors told me that I had a form of breast cancer with a poor prognosis, the very last thing I thought about was my job or the other many 'things' I was involved in. While much of what I was doing was for good reason, it was not necessary and had completely "filled my plate". I believe that true temperance is staying away from anything that is harmful and not overdoing anything that is good. It was time to make some changes. I really wanted to do all I could to be around for my husband and son, who were REALLY more important to me than anything else in this world.

Many times we over-commit ourselves to good things and feel it through stress, insomnia, short tempers, panic attacks, indigestion, headaches, etc. We then complicate matters by eating and drinking things that we know do absolutely nothing positive for building our body temples. Know when to say **NO** and when to say **WHEN**!! Even too much of a good thing can sometimes be harmful. Choose to set limits, and stick to them. (I have learned how to say no and enjoy it!) It will help to keep your life in better balance and your STRESS level down.

Look at the following chart. Take stock of the "things" you are doing. List what you are currently doing/responsible for doing? How much of what you are doing is really enhancing your life?

Is there balance in your life? Is there something(s) that needs changing? What will you do to make the changes?   When will you begin to make the needed changes?

THIS IS MY LIFE

DIET	HOME	JOB	FAMILY	CHURCH	CIVIC	SELF	GOD

WATER

"And, let him that is athirst come. And whosoever will, let him take the water of life freely." Revelation 22:17

> *I have never really had a problem drinking water. Six to eight cups per day are what is recommended. My son, Ivey, however, prefers liquids that are colored and sweetened. One day after he had played basketball, he came in and went straight to the refrigerator and proceeded to pour a large glass of juice. "No you may not!" I said. "But Mommy, I am sweating because I played so hard," he responded. "Are you sweating juice?" I asked him. This led to a wonderful discussion on the benefits of water and needless to say, now he drinks water without the big fight.*

Since our bodies are about three-fourths water, it is vitally important to keep giving it a fresh supply. Yes, you can drink other liquids but, there is nothing quite like water to restore the body. Drink some water today. You need at least 8 eight ounce glasses every single day. If you don't drink until you are thirsty, you are already becoming dehydrated.

Did you know what water does?

1. Carries body chemicals throughout the body system
2. Aids in the digestion of food (should be taken at least ½ hour before or after a meal so it won't interfere with digestion.)
3. Keeps all moving body parts lubricated.
4. Purifies the blood.
5. Invigorates body organs.
6. Regulates the body temperature.

7. Contributes to proper bowel elimination.

8. Aids in resisting diseases.

Guess what it can do on the outside of the body?

A **hot water treatment** followed by a cold water application increases the red blood cells from 20-35%. These red blood cells clean and nourish the body. But even more important, the white blood cells, which fight infections, are increased from 200-300% after a hot and cold water treatment. What a blessing!

The effect of a **cold water treatment**, temperature of the water below 85 degrees, is an instant contraction of the small arteries. A brief application of cold water produces a momentary contraction followed by relaxation and an increase in the blood supply to the specific area.

The effect of a **hot water treatment**, temperature of the water higher than 98 degrees, will increase the circulation. Hot baths are extremely stimulating to the system.

The effects of a **warm water treatment**, temperature of the water between 85 and 92 degrees are mild and soothing. The warm bath increases the action of the skin through absorption and perspiration.

Because water applied externally has all of these wonderful characteristics, we can identify the following healthful uses of water:

1. Toxins in the system are destroyed and the elimination of these toxins is increased.

2. Due to an increase in circulation and a stimulating effect on the eliminating organs, overall elimination is greatly increased.

3. Due to an increase in circulation, the body's metabolism and the formation of red and white blood cells is increased.

4. There is relief from pain and irritation.

I have personally used water (hydrotherapy) in my new way of life. Everyday, I take a hot and cold shower. This is especially helpful to me in the wintertime as it helps to reduce my risk of getting the flu.

Another treatment I've used is the hot and cold sitz baths. Before my diagnosis, I had suffered for years with abnormal periods, clotting, fibroids, anemia, anovulatory cycles, and had several surgeries to address uterine polyps. (Joann, my friend, said I was like the woman in the Bible with the issue of blood). My gynecologist offered the pill to "normalize" the hormone levels, but I refused. After the diagnosis and changing my way of life, all of those problems disappeared. I noticed, however, that whenever I was under stress, some of the old problems resurfaced.

I discovered that the hot and cold sitz baths worked wonders and I could feel immediate results. I bought 2 plastic tubs, big enough to sit in, and placed them in my bathtub. I fill one with cold water and two trays of ice. The other I fill with hot water. After putting on a bathing suit (the water doesn't shock your skin in the tender areas when covered), I sit in the hot water first for about 3-4 minutes and then the cold for about 1 minute. As the hot water starts to feel cool I add more hot water. I do this contrast about 5-6 times. After drying myself, I briskly rub my tummy, lower back and thighs with a COLD cloth that has been wet and wrung out. Then, I rest (in bed, on sofa) for about 30 minutes afterwards. I start the treatment the week after my period ends, doing it 5 times that week, three times the second week and twice the third week. I did this for three months and have seen dramatic results within that time period.

My brother, who had neuropathy problems was also benefitted by a similar treatment.

AIR

"And the Lord God formed man of the dust of the ground, and breathed into his nostrils, the *Breath of Life* and man became a living soul." Genesis 2:7

You can live without food and water for a lot longer than you do air. It is when God breathed air into man, that he LIVED! My family now understands the true benefits of air. We try to spend lots of time outdoors and keep some windows in our home open 24-hours a day, 7 days a week.

The benefits that are received from having a constant supply of pure, fresh air are:

1. Fresh air purifies the blood, imparts to it a bright color, and sends the blood, a life giving current to every part of the body.

2. Air soothes the nerves, stimulates appetite, helps digestion and induces sound, refreshing sleep.

3. Oxygen electrifies the whole system, causes the body to be strong and healthy, and will refresh the system.

4. Air invigorates the vital organs and aids the system in getting rid of an accumulation of impurities.

5. Pure air brings life to the skin, as for a lack of air the skin nearly dies.

6. But most important, air has a decided influence on the mind, imparting a degree of composure and serenity.

7. Some specific problems that are greatly benefitted by having an abundance of fresh air are: fevers, colds, and lung diseases.

Yielding To Divine Power

"I know the plans I have for you, plans to prosper you and not to harm you, plans to give you hope and a good future."
Jeremiah 29:11 (New International Version)

With the world as crazy as it is, so many of us have adopted the "I've got to do all this to take care of myself (family). I'd better look out for myself (family), and if you get in my way, that's too bad for you" attitude. This leads to overwork, overeating, overachieving, overweight, stress, regret, disregard for others, etc. After my diagnosis, I fully realized that God was in charge of everything. I really needed to trust Him to provide EVERYTHING for me. When we develop a childlike trust in God, we are able to find contentment in the midst of whatever situation we may face. He made us. He knows exactly what's ahead. By staying in touch with Him, we can know His plan for our lives and depend on Him to help us fulfill that plan. Science is confirming, that those who have a regular spiritual factor in their lives face life without as much stress, have less disease, heal better, and live longer. I spend at least 30 minutes per day in communion with God.

Whenever you are faced with a trying situation - illness, debt, marital problems, loneliness, depression, substance abuse/addiction, etc., believe that God has the answer and the power to heal that situation. **ANYTIME** we ask to be rescued from bad habits, He offers it freely.

When we go to Him and ask for other things, and ask that His will be done, we are in effect saying, Lord, I know what You **can** do, and this is what I want You to do for me. But, if it is not

66

Your will, I accept Your will as best for me. When we release control to Him, we receive a peace that passes all understanding. We can walk away knowing that He will do what is best for me, and it will happen when it is best for me. We will trust that He is able to do "exceedingly, abundantly above all that we could ask or think" (Ephesians 3:19). And when our request for healing involves confession and repentance of some behavior that contributed to us getting where we are, we must stop the behavior and walk in a newness of life.

When I realized that God had indeed spared my life, I was happy to share His mercy with others who were going through the same thing. I wanted **everyone** to have the same outcome I did. I had to accept, very painfully, that sometimes, some of us will die. **BUT**, when we realize that death is not the end, we have hope. After watching my father die, I was convinced that death with hope is so much better than life with suffering. For daddy, healing will come at the resurrection.

So, when the question surfaces, "Donna, what if the cancer returns and you worsen and die? What then?" My answer is this, "Because I believe that when God heals you it is thorough and complete, I am accepting this gift of healing. As long as I am following the will of my heavenly Father, "no weapon formed against me, shall prosper,"(Isaiah 54: 17) and that includes death. When He decides that I have completed all that He has put me on earth to do, then I can go to my grave, with the hope of the resurrection. And when He comes back to end the misery of this place called earth, I will rise again and be welcomed into eternal life. How do I know this? I have read His promises to me.
My Bible tells me:
*It's appointed unto all men once to die. (Hebrews 9:27) Not one

of the people that Jesus healed when He was on earth is alive today.

*The living know that they shall die, but the dead know not anything. (Ecclesiastes 9:5)

*Jesus compares death to a sleep. (John 11:11)

*And when one dies, his breath goeth forth, he returneth to the earth and in that very day his thoughts perish. (Psalm 146:4)

*Blessed are the dead which die in the Lord from henceforth: that they may rest from their labours and their works do follow them. (Revelation 14:13)

*Be thou faithful unto death, and I will give you a crown of life. (Revelation 2:10)

*We shall not all sleep, but we shall be changed....O death, where is thy sting, O grave where is thy victory? (1 Corinthians 15:51-55)

*But I would not have you to be ignorant, brethren, concerning them which are asleep, that ye sorrow not, even as others which have no hope. For if we believe that Jesus died and rose again, even so them also which sleep in Jesus will God bring with him. For this we say unto you by the word of the Lord that we which are live and remain unto the coming of the Lord shall not prevent them which are asleep. For the Lord himself shall descend from heaven with a shout, with the voice of the archangel, and with the trump of God: and the dead in Christ shall rise first. Then we which are alive and remain shall be caught up together with them in the clouds to meet the Lord in the air; and so shall we ever be with the Lord.

(1 Thessalonians 4:13-18)

*And I saw a new heaven and a new earth...

And there shall be no more **death**, neither **sorrow,** nor **crying,** nor **tears,**

for the former things are passed away. (Revelation 21:1,4)

There's gonna be a great reunion, real soon.

I'll get to see Daddy, Aunt Priss,

Marquita, Rashida, Joanie, Gretchen, Christi,

Gramma Hazel, Pop

and a whole lot of other folks!

And, **then** I will *REALLY* have

Somethin' to Shout About!!!!!

Glory, Hallelujah!!

You Can Shout Too!

*C*ancer, heart disease, diabetes, stroke, obesity, chronic fatigue, hypertension, digestive tract problems, arthritis, allergies, asthma, depression, nicotine and caffeine addiction, anxiety, auto-immune diseases, upper respiratory diseases, and chronic headache plague our nation. Among people of color, specifically African-Americans, the burden of morbidity and mortality from these diseases is disproportionately higher when compared to the general population. Much of what is done to address these diseases is **symptom-focused** instead of **cause-focused.** While modern medicine has made great strides in being able to take care of the human body, many of us can do far more for our *own* health than anybody else can. I have yet to see anyone whose health cannot be affected for the better by making positive lifestyle choices.

If you want to shout too, make a commitment to choosing those *lifestyle habits* that will help you to be in "good health". It really is the **BEST WAY!** There are no products. It's not expensive. It's equal opportunity. It's a way of life. It's endorsed by the Great Physician. Don't put it off another minute. Do it today!!

Beloved, I wish above all things, that thou mayest prosper and be in good health, even as thy soul prospereth. 3 John 2

BEST WAY

Here is the BEST WAY to start your new lifestyle. By practicing the *Principles for Better Health*, you're sure to see an improvement in your health.

	SUNDAY	MONDAY	TUESDAY	WEDNESDAY	THURSDAY	FRIDAY	SATURDAY
BEDTIME							
EXERCISE							
SUNSHINE							
SIMPLE DIET							
TEMPERANCE							
WATER							
AIR							
YIELD TO DIVINE POWER							

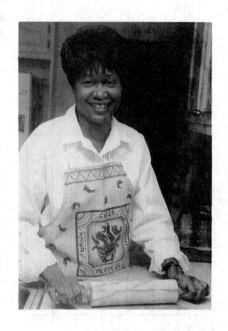

Welcome to Donna's Kitchen!

HERE'S WHAT'S COOKIN'

IN DONNA'S KITCHEN

Here's What's Cookin' in Donna's Kitchen

When I was growing up, my mom and dad were always cooking something good for us to eat. Daddy was actually the most creative cook of the two. But he would always leave the kitchen in a BIG mess. Mommy, however, gave me the principles of cooking. At age 10, I cooked my first dinner. I was so proud.

One day, during my sophomore year in high school, I had made plans to hang out with my friends. As I was explaining my plans to my mom, she promptly burst my bubble and said that on that day I was going to learn to bake bread. Bake bread!! No way!! I was hanging out. I quickly went in search of my daddy, in the hope that **he** could convince her to let me go. It was not to be.

With a major teenage attitude, I joined mommy in the kitchen for my bread baking lesson. The bread was a total success. And, needless to say, that day was a real turning point in my life. I eventually got to hang out with my friends. But mommy helped me to develop a love of cooking.

As a matter of fact, when I was in college, my then boyfriend's dorm resident assistant said that I was the first young lady he had met that cooked like an old woman! My husband (who was won over by a carrot cake and yeast rolls) and son are now my best critics, and I appreciate so much their allowing me to practice on them!

After my diagnosis, I decided to include diet as a large part of my new way of life. Because of my choice to adopt a vegan vegetarian diet, I purposed to create some tasty dishes for my family and friends, including the meat-eating ones. This is not an end all collection of **everything** you need to know about adding more plant foods to your diet. Nor is it all you can possibly do with vegan, vegetarian cooking. What follows is a number of those recipes that I have prepared for family, friends and cooking classes. They are foods that I am familiar with, and enjoy preparing. Some recipes are original, others are modifications of favorites and some I found and am sharing because we enjoy them. My friend Joann thinks I should already be working on the second collection of recipes. We'll see! Hope you enjoy these and the health tips. If something doesn't taste like you thought it would, get in that kitchen and experiment! Make them appealing to **your** family and friends.

Vegetarianism! The Best Way to Eat

Scientific evidence is mounting that a plant-based dietary is the best route to take if you are trying to improve your health. Often, a person's exposure to a plant-based diet will determine how vegetarian he or she becomes. It's a good idea to take people where they are and give them something better. Part of the reason I was determined to come up with some *tasty* vegetarian dishes, was so that people wouldn't have an excuse once they tasted it. Of the many people who have come to our classes, doubtful at first to taste the samples, all of them are able to enjoy something. And when they leave, they want to know when the next cooking class is.

So what really is a vegetarian? Actually, its a person who subsists on plant foods. Vegetarians do **not** eat chicken and fish. Within the broad category of vegetarian there are several types:

Lacto Vegetarian: One who eats plant products and milk products.

Ovo Vegetarian: One who eats plant products and egg products.

Lacto-Ovo Vegetarian: One who eats plant foods and milk and egg products.

Vegan Vegetarian: One who eats plant foods ONLY

Until my diagnosis, I had been a lacto-ovo vegetarian. I am sure I ate my and someone else's share of milk, milk products, cheese and cheese products. I loved french fries, and could bake a mean pound cake. Reese's peanut butter and bubble gum ice creams were my favorite. Unfortunately, all of those delicious tasting foods were high in fat and sugar and other stimulating/irritating substances that are known to be disease-promoting instead of health-promoting. Fortunately, there are delicious foods that you can use to replace them. There are a lot of new options on the market for the person who needs to have some things already prepared. Enjoy the following tips on diet, the list of recommended foods you can use in the transition and recipes for the *best diet* in the world!!!

BENEFITS OF BREAKFAST

The importance of breakfast has been documented many times in the medical literature. But more importantly the Word of God indicates that God would have His children eat a good breakfast every day. (Exodus 16:8; 1 Kings 17:6) A few of the known benefits of a good breakfast:

*Men who ate a good breakfast regularly had a 40% lower risk of dying than those who skipped breakfast. Women who ate a good breakfast had a 30% lower risk.

*Regular good breakfasts make a significant contribution to how people perceive their well-being. We feel better when we get in the habit of eating a good breakfast.

*Those who ate a good high complex carbohydrate breakfast had more energy, less fatigue and less sleepiness than those who skipped breakfast. A high protein breakfast on the other hand, though it consisted of the same number of calories caused more fatigue and sleepiness.

*Skipping breakfast results in a transient hunger that has affected behavior. This causes decreased attentiveness, hyperactivity and irritability.

*School performance was better in those who ate breakfast than those who did not eat breakfast.

*Blood cholesterol levels are lowest among adults eating a good breakfast that includes a high-fiber cereal. Those who skipped breakfast had the highest cholesterol levels.

*Those who eat a good breakfast are more likely to eat good meals the rest of the day.

What Constitutes a Good Breakfast?

A high complex carbohydrate diet is best. This includes whole grains and fruits. Adequate protein is also very important. This can best be accomplished with a whole grain breakfast cereal, soy or skim milk, one or two pieces of fresh, canned or dried fruit and a couple pieces of 100% whole grain toast. **NOT** the typical sugar-laden, high-fat, empty calorie foods we usually eat.

David L. Moore, M.D.

FEELING A LITTLE STRESSED?
It could be something you ate!!!
Stimulating foods wreak havoc on the body.
Check out the list below.

The following foods and food habits can be irritating to the stomach and the digestive system. When that system is upset, we often experience symptoms such as: headache, stomachache, gas, belching, inability to concentrate, inability to relax, tiredness, anxiousness, **STRESS!!!**☺☹ All of which can lead to a number of diseases.

1.   Hot pepper, black or red and spices-ginger, cinnamon, cloves, nutmeg.

2.   Vinegar and anything made with vinegar (which is but decayed, fermented apples)-pickles, mayonnaise, salad dressing, mustard, catsup, etc.

3.   Foods having a fermenting, putrifying or rotting phase in processing, such as sauerkraut, cheese, soy sauce and similar products.

4.   Baking soda, baking powder products, including commercial salted crackers, all commercial cookies, doughnuts and other bakery items.

5.   Caffeine (coffee, tea, colas, chocolate), nicotine, theobromine (from chocolate)

6.   Drinking with meals. Digestion and stomach emptying are both delayed. Stagnation in the stomach is one of the commonest causes of ulcers and gastritis. Milk contains much lactose, the milk sugar that promotes fermentation and production of irritating toxic chemicals. Milk is the cause of more sensitivity to food than any other food item.

7. Late evening meals.

8. Eating too much. Most people could get by very well with one-half or two-thirds less than they presently eat.

9. Chewing too little. Eating too fast. Bites too large.

10. Foods rich with refined sugar, refined oils, vitamin and mineral preparations, or concentrated proteins such as heavy meat substitutes and dried milk products The more concentrated the food, the more likely to irritate the stomach.

11. Eating fruits and vegetables at the same meal. Foods that contain combinations of milk and eggs, milk and sugar, or eggs and sugar.

12. Unripe or overripe fruit.

13. Foods that are taken while they are too hot or too cold.

14. Crowding meals closer together than five hours.

THOSE WONDERFUL COOKING HERBS

While it is easy to cook the way we are used to, using ingredients that add taste and health benefit is the BEST WAY to go. I now grow my own herbs.

PARSLEY	Parsley contains a substance that prevents the multiplication of tumor cells. It relieves gas, stimulates normal activity of the digestive system and freshens breath. Helps bladder, kidney, liver, lung, stomach and thyroid function. Good for high blood pressure and indigestion.	Vegetables, main dishes, soups, salads, breath freshener
SAGE	One of the most valued herbs of antiquity, sage is highly antiseptic, excellent remedy for colds, fevers, sore throats; relieves tonsilitis, bronchitis, asthma, sinusitis. Has a tonic effect upon the female reproductive tract; also estrogenic and is excellent for menopausal problems. It helps to reduce the harmful effects of free radicals.	Vegetables, soups, main dishes, breads, quiches, scrambled tofu, gravies
ROSEMARY	Rosemary contains oils which are antiseptic, with antibacterial and antifungal proper which enhance the function of the immune system. By increasing circulation to the skin, rosemary causes sweating and makes a good remedy to bring down fevers. It stimulates digestion, relieves gas, stimulates liver and gallbladder function. It is a powerful antioxidant.	Cornbread dressing, vegetables, soups
THYME	A powerful antiseptic. It enhances the immune system's fight against bacterial, viral and fungal infections, especially in the respiratory, digestive and genitourinary system such as colds, coughs, flu, gastroenteritis, candida and cystitis. It has a relaxing effect on the bronchial tubes; and acts as an expectorant by increasing the production of fluid mucous and shifting phlegm. Thyme is a liver tonic, stimulating the digestive system.	Vegetables, breads, main dishes, soups, rice dishes, pastas, salads, gravies

THOSE WONDERFUL COOKING HERBS

While it is easy to cook the way we are used to, using ingredients that add taste and health benefit is the BEST WAY to go. I now grow my own herbs.

GARLIC	Garlic is an effective remedy against bacterial, fungal, viral and parasitic infections. It contains many sulfur compounds which give it its marvelous healing properties. Contains the substance *allicin* which has been shown to be more powerful than penicillin and tetracycline. It detoxifies the body and protects against infection by enhancing the immune function (excellent for AIDS patients). It lowers blood pressure and blood lipid levels and improves circulation. Aids in the treatment of arteriosclerosis, arthritis, asthma, cancer (anti-tumor forming), circulatory problems, colds and flu, digestive problems, sinusitis, yeast infections.	Vegetables, soups, salads, main dishes, scrambled tofu. Medicinal teas
DILL	Dill has an antispasmodic action, relieving spasm in the digestive tract. It enhances digestion, relieves indigestion, nausea, constipation, hiccoughs. It induces sleep in babies and children; increases milk supply in breast-feeding mothers; relieves painful periods. Can be used externally in warming lineaments to increase circulation in the limbs and to sooth muscular tension and joint pain.	Vegetables, soups, breads, salad dressings
PEPPERMINT	Antiseptic, antibacterial, antiparasitic, antifungal, antiviral, antispasmodic, decongestant. Induces heat and causes sweating, relieves stuffiness. A good general tonic, has excellent cooling effect. Good local application to relieve pain-inflamed joints in arthritis/gout, headache. Reduces inflammation in digestive tract relieving stomach aches, colic, gas, heartburn, indigestion, hiccoughs, nausea, vomiting, travel sickness. Cleanses the liver and gallbladder.	Salads/dressings, fruits, vegetables, beverages Medicinal teas

WHEN SUGAR TURNS SOUR!

MANY OF US "TREAT" OURSELVES TO SUGAR- - SOMETIMES - - A SLICE OF MAMA'S APPLE PIE, A DOUBLE FUDGE SUNDAE WITH NUTS, HOLIDAY CANDIES, HOMEMADE POUND CAKE. WHILE IT TASTES GOOD GOING DOWN, YOU MAY NOT REALIZE WHAT IT DOES TO YOUR BODY ONCE IT GETS INSIDE. CONSIDER THESE FACTS

FACT Too much sugar depletes the body of B vitamins. B vitamins are essential for healthy nerves. A depletion of B vitamins lowers our resistance to infection and makes us irritable and depressed.

FACT Too much sugar increases the blood fat levels and tends to clog the arteries. This lowers the body's resistance to disease. Sugar plays a significant role in the buildup of cholesterol.

FACT Too much sugar contributes to tooth decay, because it slows the fluid flow through the tiny canals of the teeth. The teeth lose their resistance to viral and bacterial invasion and decay results.

FACT Rich, heavy desserts cause irritation of the stomach, mental dullness, and obesity. Natural sweets can satisfy the "sweet tooth" while furnishing vitamins and minerals.

FACT Too much sugar weakens the white blood cells, which furnish our mainline of defense against invading germs. One white cell can normally attack and destroy 14 invading germs. After eating an excess of sugar, this capability is reduced dramatically.

COMMON SWEETS	ALTERNATIVES
Syrup	Fruit Sauce
Ice Cream	Smoothies
Jams	Fruit Spreads
Soft Drinks	Water (between meals)
Candy	Dried Fruit
Pastries	Fruit Breads
Cookies	Wholesome cookies

SUGAR'S EFFECT ON WHITE BLOOD CELLS

Every winter, families fight bouts with colds and flu. I have always wondered how that could be since during winter, which is the cold season, the number of harmful germs should actually be reduced. The first winter after my family changed our diets, we sailed through the cold and flu season without getting sick. After doing some investigation, I discovered some rather interesting information. A number of different studies had been conducted by researchers testing the effect of sugar consumption on the white blood cells ability to fight disease. (One of my professors from Loma Linda University, Dr. Albert Sanchez, was involved in some of the research). These scientists noticed that the more sugar that was consumed, the less able white blood cells were able to fight infection. The effects of the sugar on the white blood cells last a while.

I got to thinking and realized that from Halloween to Valentine's Day, we overdose on sugar. We inhibit our body's ability to fight disease and end up getting sick. The following chart shows how disabled the white cells actually become. **Note,** one banana split **OR** 2-12 ounce soft drinks easily contributes 24 teaspoons of sugar. What about all that other yummy stuff we eat over the winter holiday season!?!?!? List what you usually eat. Could this be why you get sick?

_____

_____

_____

_____

_____

Amount of Sugar Eaten at One Time by Average Adult in Teaspoons	Number of Bacteria Destroyed by Each White Blood Cell	Percent Decrease in Ability to Destroy Bacteria
No Sugar	14 Bacteria	0%
6 Teaspoons	10 Bacteria	25%
12 Teaspoons	5.5 Bacteria	60%
18 Teaspoons	2 Bacteria	85%
24 Teaspoons	1 Bacteria	92%

SUGGESTIONS FOR CONTROLLING SUGAR INTAKE

1. **DO NOT** put sugar on the table. Try using raisins, dates, or some other fruit for a natural sweetener instead of sugar.

2. Use dark brown sugar, molasses, honey and dried fruits with as little white sugar as possible. Be sparing with ALL concentrated sweets.

3. When serving a dessert high in calories, plan for it in the meal by serving less calories in the main part of the meal.

4. Build up a supply of recipes using little or no sugar. In many desserts the quantity of sugar used can be cut in half and the dessert will be acceptable.

5. Buy NO SUGAR COATED BREAKFAST FOOD!! (cereals, pastries, donuts, etc.)

6. Avoid desserts that use large quantities of milk, sugar and eggs together (like puddings).

7. Learn to make desserts without the use of baking soda. It is an irritant to the digestive tract and destroys vitamins.

8. Let desserts be a special treat--not served *every* day of the week!

9. Use unsweetened fruit juices instead of heavily sugared ones.

10. Many fruit recipes do not need any sugar at all. Use more fresh fruit and frozen fruit without added or large

amounts of sugar added. When buying canned fruit, choose the one with *light syrup* instead of **heavy syrup**. Well prepared fruit dishes can replace concentrated, refined sweets that we so freely eat.

11.   Take sweet foods chiefly at the end of a meal.

12.   Do not eat candy or other sweets between meals.

13.   Avoid large amounts of sugar and milk in combination (ice cream). In the stomach, they cause fermentation.

14.   Keep the total amount of sugar in the diet low, and take only small amounts of concentrated sweets.

WHAT!!! NO CHOCOLATE? WHY NOT??

Here is a table designed to help you evaluate chocolate and it's suitability as a food compared to carob. Make your decision based on **FACTS** AND NOT ON **TASTE AND HABITS** ALONE.

CHOCOLATE	CAROB
Methylxanthines: are contributing factors in breast cancer and possibly prostate cancer. Caffeine is a methylxanthine. It is wise to discontinue the use of coffee, tea, colas, chocolate and all forms of methylxanthines.	No methylxanthines
Tannin: is present in all brands of cocoa from which chocolate is made and can have harmful effects on the mucous membranes of the digestive tract.	No tannins
Theobromine: causes headaches, central nervous system irritation, itching, depression, anxiety and fibrocystic disease of the breast.	No theobromine
Sugar: in large amounts is required to mask the bitter flavor and make it palatable.	**Naturally sweet**
Fat: makes up a minimum of 50% of chocolate's calories. Oil, cream or milk is often added which makes it extremely rich, heavy , oily and difficult to digest.	**Low** in fat (about 2% of its calories)
Contamination: often occurs during the processing of cocoa beans. The bean pods are left in piles outdoors to ferment for several days. Fermentation is essential to develop the chocolate flavor. Aflatoxins, which are cancer promoting toxins produced by molds, are produced in the beans. In addition, insects, rodents and small animals may make nests in the piles. Though the beans are later cleaned, roasted and shelled, contaminants may be present. The US Department of Health and Human Services does allow for some contamination in chocolate from "insects, rodents, and other natural contaminants."	No fermentation necessary; no known allergic reactions Source: Weimar's NEWSTART Lifestyle Cookbook

Biblical Reference:
Matthew 3:4 And the same John had his raiment of camel's hair, and a leathern girdle about his loins. And his meat was locusts **(locust bean)** and wild honey

Mark 1:6 And John was clothed with camel's hair, and with a girdle of skin about his loins; and he did eat locusts **(locust bean)** and wild honey.

HOW SWEET IT IS OR ISN'T!!

"Hidden" sugar comprises 76% of our sugar intake. Only 24% is added in the home--the rest is added by the food and beverage industry. The consumer is confronted by a wide variety of sugars and other nutritive sweeteners, and there is no significant difference in the amount of calories each provides. A brief explanation of the more common sugars and sweeteners is listed on the left. On the right is a list of alternatives to refined sugar.

Brown sugar: Consists of sugar crystals contained in molasses syrup with natural flavor and color. Some refiners make brown sugar by simply adding syrup to refined white sugar in a mixer. It is 91-96% sucrose.

Corn Syrups: Produced by the action of enzymes and/or acids on cornstarch. High fructose corn syrup comes from corn.

Dextrose: Also known as glucose or corn sugar. Made commercially from starch by the action of heat and acids or enzymes. Often sold blended with regular sugar.

Fructose: Known as fruit sugar, it occurs naturally in many fruits. Also known as levulose, it is a commercial sugar considerably sweeter than sucrose, although its sweetness depends on its physical form and how it is used in cooking.

Maltitol, Mannitol, Sorbitol, Xylitol: Sugar alcohols or pollyols, which occur naturally in fruits but are commercially produced from such sources such sources as dextrose. Xylitol is a sugar alcohol made from a part of birch trees.

Sucrose: Obtained in crystalline from cane and beets; a double sugar or disaccharide composed of two simple sugars - glucose and fructose. It is about 99.9% pure and is sold in either granulated or powdered form.

Barley Malt: A wholesome, nutritious, complex sweetener. It is made by partially sprouting barley grain, drying the sprouts, then grinding them into a fine flour. It is more nutritious than white sugar.

Blackstrap Molasses: Made from sugarcane. It is more nutritious than white sugar.

Brown Rice Syrup: Made from malted brown rice, which has been **fermented**. Not recommended.

Date Sugar: Dried dates ground until semi-fine. An excellent substitute for white sugar. Dates are very high in sucrose and dextrose, yet high in mineral salts, Vitamins A, B, C and fiber.

Evaporated Cane Juice: Tan to brown in appearance; coarse, granulated solid obtained from evaporation of sugarcane juice.

Fruit Juice Concentrates: Minimally processed. Made by removing moisture from natural juices.

Honey: An invert sugar formed by an enzyme from nectar gathered by bees. Composition and flavor depend on the source of the nectar. It is more nutritious than white sugar and is sweeter.

Maple Syrup: Made from the sap of the maple tree. More nutritious than white sugar, good source of calcium.

Source: Weimar New Start Lifestyle Cookbook

GET RID OF THE FAT!!

FRIED CHICKEN, FRENCH FRIES, POTATO CHIPS, POUND CAKE, ICE CREAM, CHOCOLATE CANDY, CHEESE, MACARONI AND CHEESE, PIZZA, DONUTS, PASTRIES, CHICKEN WINGS, LUNCH MEAT, CREAMY SALAD DRESSINGS, BACON, WHOPPER, BIG MAC, WHOLE MILK, COLLARDS AND BLACK EYE PEAS COOKED IN FAT BACK, CRACKLIN' BREAD. THEY ALL DO TASTE GOOD GOING DOWN. PART OF THE REASON THAT THEY DO IS BECAUSE FAT ADDS FLAVOR. IT ALSO WREAKS HAVOC ON OUR BODIES AND INCREASES OUR RISK FOR A NUMBER OF DISEASES.

FACT Fat has 2 1/4 times the amount of calories of either carbohydrates and protein per unit weight. **Carbohydrates-4 calories/gram, Proteins-4 calories/gram, Fat-9 calories/gram.**

FACT Fat is one of the MAJOR causes of obesity.

FACT High fat intake is associated with diabetes and many types of cancer, including breast, prostate and colon.

FACT High fat intake distorts the normal functions of white blood cells, particularly T & B lymphocytes.

FACT High fat in the diet is associated with gall bladder disease and gallstones.

FACT High fat intake particularly saturated fat is associated with heart disease.

COMMONLY USED FATS	ALTERNATIVES
Lard	Corn oil
Meat Drippings	Vegetable Oil blend
Butter	Vegetable Oil margarine
Canned Vegetable Shortening	Olive Oil
Fat Back	Canola Oil
Ham Hocks	Olives
Bacon	Nuts in Moderation
Mayonnaise/Salad Dressings	Sunflower Oil
Cheese	Tofu

We must reduce the use of FAT in our diets to enjoy optimal health!

NO DAIRY? WHAT ABOUT CALCIUM?
Plant Sources of Calcium

Vegetables, 1 cup	mg
Collards	357
Turnip Greens	249
Kale	179
Broccoli Pieces	177
Okra	176
Mustard Greens	104

Cooked Beans, 1 c.	
Soybeans	131
Navy	128
Pinto	86
Garbanzos	80
Black-eyed Peas	106
Lentils	37

Dried Fruits	
Figs, 3 large	78
Currants ½ cup	62
Pitted Dates, ½ cup	58
Apricots, ½ cup	50
Raisins, 2 oz	36
Prunes, ½ cup	30

Others	Mg
Fortified Soy Milk, 1 cup	100-500
Tofu/calcium salts	300
Blackstrap Molasses, 1 T.	137
Tahini, ½ oz	115
Tofu, 4 oz	110
Almonds, 1 oz	75
Sweet Potato, 1 med.	72
Medium Orange, 1	55
Bread, 2 slices	45

Dairy Prod. Comparison	
Fruit flavored/low fat Yogurt	
8 oz/added milk solids	345
Low-fat milk, 1 cup	300
Cheddar Cheese, 1 oz	204
Low-fat Cottage Cheese ½ cup	77

Reference:

Bowes & Church's - Food Values of Portions Commonly Used, edited by Jean A.T. Pennington, Ph.D, RD, 15th Edition, 1989

Nutrition for the Eighties by Winston J. Craig, PhD, RD, 1992

What are my Calcium Needs?

The recommended dietary allowance (RDA) for the average adult is
 800 mg. per day.

Am I really getting what I need?
Do the Math!!

BREAKFAST

granola	
soy milk, 1 cup	250 mg
raisins 2 oz	36
bread, 2 slices	45
medium orange	55

TOTAL

LUNCH

black-eyed peas, 1 cup	106
rice	
collard greens, 1½ cup	535
sweet potato, 1 medium	72
cornbread, 1 piece	

TOTAL

SUPPER

watermelon, 2 pieces	72
1" x 10"	

TOTAL

GRAND TOTAL

WHAT'S A PHYTOCHEMICAL?

Phytochemicals are natural chemicals found **ONLY** in plant foods. They **cannot** be obtained from **any animal** products - flesh, milk, cheese, eggs, fat, ice cream, etc.

While I was at Wildwood, I discovered first hand that these phytochemicals are being investigated by the National Cancer Institute and I needed to eat plenty of the foods in which they were found to help in reducing my risk of a reoccurrence. I was told that the deeply colored fruits like blueberries, strawberries, raspberries, and grapes had been shown to starve cancer cells of oxygen, thus causing their death. Citrus fruits, specifically lemons, oranges, and grapefruits contained substances that were anti-tumor forming. And, garlic and onions had the same properties. I was stunned!!!

Using the information I had learned at Wildwood, I went on a personal search of my own and discovered the following general information.

Phytochemicals are generally classified into several major categories. Each category is comprised of specific plant chemicals that scientists have isolated according to their effect on the body. Not only do these foods benefit cancer, but they are beneficial in other chronic diseases as well. One category of phytochemical is actually the same name (protease inhibitors) as a classification of drugs used to treat HIV/AIDS.

At Lifestyle Principles, we see patients that present variations of all the major chronic diseases. Those who have included a plant-based diet in their new way of life are being benefitted greatly. It's no wonder! This is the exact same diet laid out for us by our Creator at the beginning of time. "Behold I have given you every **herb bearing seed**, which is upon the face of all the earth, and every tree, in the which is the **fruit of a tree yielding seed;** to you it shall be for **MEAT**." (Genesis 1:29) Records indicate that the people who ate this diet lived easily over 900 years. Sounds like a plan to me!!

PHYTOCHEMICALS		
CLASS	FUNCTION	SOURCE
Allium Compounds	anti-cancer, anti-blood clotting, helps lower cholesterol/blood pressure	garlic, onions, chives, leeks, shallots
Glucosinolate Compounds	anti-cancer, anti-oxidant, anti-tumor growth, blocks carcinogens	mustard, kale, turnips, cabbage, broccoli, cauliflower
Indoles	anti-cancer, especially estrogen dependent ones	collards, turnips, kale, cabbage, cauliflower, rutabaga
Plant Polyphenols Flavonoids Phytoestrogens	anti-cancer benefits cholesterol, tri-glyceride, blood pressure levels and heart disease	fruits and vegetables beans, especially soy seeds, nuts some herbs
Terpenes	anti-cancer, immune enhancer, cell differentiation	basil, carrots, licorice, soy, oregano, thyme (to name a few)
Protease Inhibitors	anti-cancer	whole grain products, soy, legumes, seeds
Inositols	anti-cancer, cell differentiation	lima beans, all types of bran, soy , nuts
Fatty Acids	regulates prostaglandin production, immune system booster	flax/linseed, walnuts, green leafy vegetables
Plant Sterols	anti-cancer, block estrogen promotion of breast cancer activity	nuts, fruits, vegetables

Source: Wildwood Lifestyle Center

Check out Dr. Neil Nedley's book Proof Positive by Nedley Publishing in Ardmore, Oklahoma.

The National Cancer Institute

What's Up With Soy?

The soybean has been called the most "versatile" of all beans. It contains fat, carbohydrate and protein. The protein provides all eight essential amino acids. It is rich in the essential fatty acids, linoleic and linolenic and is cholesterol free.

Traditionally an Oriental food, soy and soy products have recently gained popularity because of the discovery of the important health benefits it possesses. It has been shown to have anti-cancer activity (especially breast and prostate cancer), lower high cholesterol, lower high triglycerides, prevent oxidation of LDL cholesterol, reduce menopausal symptoms (hot flashes), prevent osteoporosis, and function as a protease inhibitor.

With all these health-enhancing qualities, why aren't more people thrilled to eat soy? Probably because it is unfamiliar, and plain tofu, one of the more popular soy products, is not very appealing. When I realized the benefits of soy, I went in search of soy products. I found oil, margarine, flour, soy nuts, dairy-like products, soups, textured vegetable protein products (vege-meats) and tofu in varying textures and degrees of firmness. My family wasn't very impressed. So, I decided to substitute the products in foods we were familiar with. You will find how I used tofu, especially, in lasagne, scrambled, cheesecakes, salad dressings and in our favorite, **ice cream**, in the recipe section. Many of the soy vege-meat substitutes are highly processed and contain dairy products. We don't use a lot of them. Those that I do recommend include:

Worthington - Chickettes, Tuno, Vegetarian Burger, Multi-Grain Cutlets, Fri-Chik(has egg whites)

Loma Linda - Big Franks, Redi-Burger

Cedar Lake - Chops, Skallops

Yves Veggie Cuisine - Canadian Bacon, Pepperoni, Deli Slices, Ground Round

Light Life - Bologna, Turkey, Ham

MorningStar Farms - Vegetarian Burger Crumbles (sold in a frozen roll), Vegan Burger

Soy milk, is available under many different labels. Manufacturers have really been very creative in imitating dairy milk. Here in Atlanta, we are fortunate to have several farmer's markets that sell the true, unadulterated, soybean milk that is simply cooked soybeans and water. I prefer this soy milk for cooking. It makes excellent cornbread! We use a commercially prepared powder for drinking and on cold cereal.

Tofu comes in a variety of textures and degrees of firmness. How you plan to use it will determine which one you choose. Here are my recommendations:

Silken - Soft or Firm
Dressings, sauces, dips, creams, ice cream, frostings
Water-packed - Soft
Puddings, pies, cheesecakes, salads
Water-packed - Firm or Extra-Firm
Slicing, marinating, grilling, stir-frying, scrambling, casseroles (lasagne)

Freezing the tofu before using it changes the texture to a "meatier" texture.

I use **soy nuts** as a garnish in my tossed salads. Include some soy products in your diet today. Your body will be grateful!

MAKING THE SWITCH

As I conduct cooking classes, I am discovering over and over again, that people will change if the recommended new foods don't sacrifice on taste. Here are some ideas to help in preserving taste for your switch to a new lifestyle, or to use in preparing foods for your vegetarian friends.

Arrowroot: White powdery substance used for thickening. I sometimes use in place of cornstarch

BAKON: This seasoning is a MUST HAVE item!! It is a smoked yeast with a natural hickory smoke flavor. I use it in all my beans, and in seasoning vegetables. Wonderful no-fat, no-cholesterol option. Available at ABC (Adventist Book Center) stores.

Bragg's Liquid Aminoes: An unfermented soy sauce substitute. Made from soybeans, high in amino acids and other minerals, and lower in sodium than soy sauce.

Carob: A wonderful substitute for chocolate, this comes from the nutritious locust bean pod. It is naturally sweet, high in vitamin A, calcium, phosphorus, potassium, iron and magnesium. Has no caffeine and much less fat. It is available in a powdered form. You can also buy it processed into carob chips. Choose the malt sweetened ones and use as you would chocolate chips.

Cashews: Classed with nuts, cashews are actually a tropical fruit. They are lower in fat than most nuts and yield a creamy sauce when blended with water, and thicken when heated. You can find them raw, roasted or as butter. When using them in a recipe for sauce, etc., use the raw ones, but wash them first as they tend to be dirty. My friend Jennifer and I sometimes substitute almonds in equal amounts when we don't have cashews on hand.

Coriander: Is the fruit of the coriander herb. Recommended as a cinnamon substitute, as cinnamon can be irritating to the digestive tract.

Emes Kosher Gel: An all vegetable gelatin containing carrageenan, locust bean gum, and cottonseed gum. Comes unsweetened and in several sweetened flavors. Use the plain for setting recipes. The flavored can be used in place of traditional gelatins. It is available at ABC stores and Jewish grocers.

Ener-G Egg Replacer: Non-dairy, powdered binding agent. It can be used as a substitute for eggs in baked goods. Follow directions on box when using it.

Featherweight Baking Powder: A baking powder that does not contain harmful aluminum or baking soda, which is a digestive tract irritant.

Flavorings: Non-alcoholic flavorings are best. The Spicery Shoppe and Frontier are two brands that I recommend and use.

Florida Crystals: Trade name for evaporated cane juice. This sugar product has not been processed as much as white sugar. I recommend its use occasionally.

Gluten Flour: The protein part of wheat. You can find it in the flour section of your grocer.

Herbs: Fresh or dried, when I realized the marvelous benefits of herbs, beyond flavoring, I planted an herb garden on my deck. Imagine cutting exactly your favorite herb in the amount you need for a dish you are preparing. I grew parsley, sage, rosemary, thyme, apple mint, basil and oregano. They were all so easy to do.

Lemon Juice: A necessary replacement for harmful vinegar, which is fermented and contains acetic acid. I buy fresh lemons, squeeze them, refrigerate the juice and use in any recipe that calls for vinegar. Limonoids, are a potent phytochemical found in citrus fruits.

McKay's Chicken Style or Beef Style Seasoning: My friend Debbie calls Chicken-Style the "Wonder" seasoning. She uses it on everything except fruit. Both seasonings are vegetarian and add a meaty flavor without the meat. The "No MSG" type is recommended. Available at ABC (Adventist Book Center) stores. Health food stores would probably order it.

Nutritional Yeast Flakes: This is an edible brewer's yeast. It comes "flaked", is yellow in color, and is the secret to making "cheez" sauces. It is high in B vitamins. Red Star is the brand I use.

PA's Pickles: These pickles are made with lemon juice instead of vinegar. They come sliced, in strips and as relish. Available at ABC (Adventist Book Center) stores.

Pimento: A heart shaped member of the pepper family. It has a sweet, mild flavor and can be added to dishes for color and/or flavor. Look for it in your grocery store on the aisle with condiments. I grew some this summer in my herb garden.

Roma: A coffee substitute made from grains. Available at ABC stores and most health food stores.

Soy Parmesan Cheese: Alternative to dairy Parmesan cheese. Three brands I am familiar with are Soya-Kass, SoyCo and Soymage. Soymage is the only one of the three that does not contain the milk protein casein.

Spectrum Spread - A non-hydrogenated spread made from vegetable oil.

Stevia: An herbal sweetener that is much sweeter than processed white sugar.

Sucanat: A granulated sugar made from organic sugar cane juice. Because it is unrefined, it still contains its original vitamins and minerals. I use it in place of brown sugar.

Turmeric: A mustard-like herb that is non-irritating to the digestive tract. It adds a wonderful color and flavor to foods. It is also being touted as having anti-cancer properties. Be careful when you start using it, it can be overpowering.

Wright's Hickory Smoke: A bottled liquid hickory smoke flavoring, that I use in barbecue sauces. This brand has no questionable ingredients.

Suggested Substitutions

For:	Use Instead:
Milk	Soy milks Rice Milks Cashew Milk
Buttermilk	Add 1 T. Lemon Juice to 1 cup non-dairy milk
Cheese	Commercial Soy Cheeses Make Cashew Cheez
Eggs, Scrambled	Scrambled Tofu
Eggs, as binder	Ener-G Egg Replacer Oats, bread crumbs, gluten flour
Chocolate	Carob
Cinnamon	Coriander
Coffee	Roma, Postum, Pero
Tea	Caffeine Free Herb Tea
Sugar	Fruit, Fruit Juice, Sucanat, Honey, Florida Crystals, Molasses
Black Pepper	Herbs
Hot Peppers	Garlic
Beef/Chicken Flavors	McKay's Chicken or Beef Style Seasoning
Turkey Wings	BAKON Seasoning

Cracklin/Bacon	Imitation Baco Bits
Vinegar	Fresh Lemon or Lime Juice
Soy Sauce	Bragg's Liquid Aminoes
Gelatin	Emes Vegetable Gelatin
Pork n' Beans	Bush's Vegetarian Baked Beans
White Rice	Brown Rice, long-grain or Instant

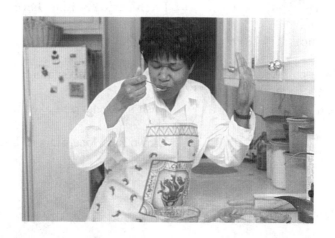

Donna tasting her peach cobbler

RECIPES

TO

SHOUT ABOUT!!

"The one who understands the art of properly preparing food, and who uses this knowledge, is worthy of higher commendation than those engaged in any other line of work. This talent should be regarded as equal in value to ten talents; for its right use has much to do with keeping the human organism in health. Because so inseparably connected with life and health, it is the most valuable of all gifts."

Counsels on Diet and Foods, p. 251

BREAKFAST

Scrambled Tofu*

2 lbs.	Firm tofu
2 T.	olive oil
1/4 c.	chopped green pepper
1/4 c.	chopped red pepper
½ c.	chopped sweet onion
2	cloves garlic, chopped
½ c.	burger crumbles, Morningstar Farms (optional)
1 T.	McKay's No MSG Chicken Style Seasoning
1 T.	Bragg's Liquid Amino (Soy Sauce Substitute)
1 T.	Nutritional yeast flakes
1/4 t.	Turmeric

Optional Seasonings: sage, parsley
Rinse, drain and crumble or strip (slice thinly in both directions)
the tofu. Heat oil in skillet, saute vegetables. Add tofu and
seasonings. Heat thoroughly and serve warm.
Serves 8

Waffle OR Pancake Batter
This is a variation of Cheryl Thomas-Peters recipe from her
book *More Choices for a Healthy Low-Fat You.*

1 pkg. silken firm tofu	1 t. alcohol-free vanilla flavoring
1 c. tofu/soy milk	3/4 c. whole wheat flour, sifted
2 T. canola oil	3/4 c. all-purpose flour, sifted
2 T. honey	1 heaping t. baking powder
1 t. lemon juice	3/4 t. salt

Place all the wet ingredients in blender and blend until smooth.
Sift together all the dry ingredients. Add the sifted dry
ingredients to the blender mixture and mix until smooth. Pour
pancake batter onto nonstick skillet and cook OR onto waffle
iron, following manufacturer's directions.

Serves 6

Pam's Pancakes or Belgian Waffles and Apple Syrup

Pam, our receptionist, makes this for her family and freezes them. They are full of whole grains and will fill you up! Try them on your family.

In a blender, blend:
2 c. hot water
½ c. cashews
1. c. oats
1 t. salt
1/3 c. sweetener

In a small bowl, dissolve:
½ t. yeast in 1/4 c. water

In a large bowl pour:
blended mixture
yeast mixture
1 ½ c. unbleached flour
½ c. whole wheat flour
1/4 c. oil
1 ½ T. vanilla
½ t. Featherweight baking powder
Mix and pour onto vegetable sprayed griddle or waffle iron.

Variations: Add fruit or nuts
            Use maple, butter or other flavorings

Apple Syrup

In a blender blend:
1-12 oz. can frozen apple juice concentrate
1-12 oz. can water
2 T. plus 2 t. cornstarch
1 t. lemon juice
½ t. coriander
Pour into pan. Cook over low heat to thicken. Stir often.

Breakfast Biscuits*

1 c.	plain unbleached flour
2/3 c	soy flour
1/3 c.	whole wheat pastry flour
1 t.	salt
4 t.	aluminum/baking soda free baking powder/Featherweight
1 T.	sugar - Florida Crystals dehydrated cane juice (optional)
6 T.	margarine - Willow Run OR 1/3 cup oil
1 c.	soy milk - your choice

Sift dry ingredients. Cut in margarine until mixture resembles corn meal. (If using oil, add to milk and stir, then add liquid ingredients to dry ingredients.) Add milk and stir quickly until mixture forms a ball. Turn onto a lightly floured board and knead gently with floured hands. Press the dough into a ball, cut in half place one half on top of the other and press down. Repeat three or four times. Then, roll out onto cutting board and cut. Place on cookie sheet and bake at 450 degrees until browned. About 12-15 minutes.

Yield: 12 servings
Variation: Use ½ unbleached and ½ whole wheat flour
Use biscuit dough to make cinnamon rolls. Filling recipe follows.

Cinnamon Roll Filling

1 c. unbleached flour
1 c. Sucanat
1 T. coriander - in place of cinnamon, which is irritating to the digestive system
1 t. salt
½ c. oil

Mix above ingredients in a bowl. Add ½ cup of optional **raisins or nuts.** Sprinkle and spread filling onto prepared pastry dough. Roll up each rectangle of dough. Slice into 1" rounds and place about 1" apart on oiled cookie sheet.

110

Banana Bread

This is a variation of *Silver Hills Guest House Cookbook* recipe.

1 c. bananas	T. Powdered Egg Replacer
1/3 c. brown sugar	½ t. salt
1/3 c. Sucanat	3/4 c. unbleached all purpose flour
1/4 c. oil	3/4 c. whole wheat pastry flour
1/2 c. soy milk	1 T. Featherweight baking powder
1 T. lemon juice	½ c. chopped nuts
1 t. coriander	

In a large bowl, mash bananas. Add other ingredients and mix until well combined. Pour bread mixture into a loaf pan that has been well sprayed. Bake for 45 minutes in a 350 degree oven. Turn out of pan and cool. Slice and serve.

Salmonette Patties

1 pound tofu, firm, crumbled
1 roll frozen, Vegetarian Tuno
1 can Vegetarian Fri-Chik (keep broth from the can)
1 medium onion, chopped
½ c. Tofutti Better Than Sour Cream
plain bread crumbs
parsley, garlic powder, paprika, McKay's Chicken Style seasoning to taste

Saute onion in a little olive oil. In a large bowl mix Tuno, grated Fri-Chik, broth, crumbled tofu, sauteed onions and sour cream. Season to taste with parsley, garlic powder, paprika, McKay's Chicken Style Seasoning. Add enough bread crumbs to form a semi-stiff mixture. Shape into patties and place on greased cookie sheet. Bake at 400 degrees until browned, turning once. Great with Italian food, grits, and gravy, as a sandwich!!

Makes about 20 patties

Bean Sausage

2 c.	cooked, drained pinto beans
1 ½ c.	bread crumbs, plain
4	EnerG egg replacers
½ c.	soy milk
1 t.	salt (optional)
3/4 t.	garlic powder
1 ½ t.	sage
½	small onion chopped fine
½ t.	Bragg's liquid amino

Homemade Gravy (optional)

Mash the beans. Mix with the egg replacer and bread crumbs. Add the remaining ingredients. Mix well. Shape the mixture into patties, place on cookie sheet that has been sprayed with non-stick spray. Bake at 400 degrees until done. Serve as is or cover with homemade gravy and let simmer about 20 minutes.

Serves 8

Oven Baked Home Fries

4 medium white potatoes (peeled, optional)
1 medium yellow onion, chopped
1 T. olive oil
2 cloves fresh garlic, minced
 salt, paprika

Wash and dice potatoes. Place oil in iron skillet. Add diced potatoes, onions, and garlic to skillet. Sprinkle with about 3/4 teaspoon salt and 1 teaspoon paprika. Stir and place uncovered in 400 degree oven. Bake till tender when pierced with a fork. Stir about every 15 minutes to avoid burning. Taste and add any additional salt, or garlic as needed before serving.

Optional: Add red and green sweet pepper
        Season with McKay's Chicken Style Seasoning,
         McCormick's Garlic and Herb Seasoning.
        Add imitation Baco-Bits during last few minutes of
         cooking
        Add BAKON for that smoked flavor

Serves 6

Homemade Granola*
I fell in love with this while at Wildwood. Here is
my version.
6 c. rolled oats
4 c. quick oats
1 c. whole wheat pastry flour
½ c. coconut
½ c. chopped nuts - almonds and sunflower seeds

Blend
½ c. water
½ c. canola oil
½ c. honey
1 T. alcohol free vanilla flavoring
1 T. alcohol free almond flavoring
1 ½ t salt
Optional: other dried fruit (I use pineapple); use maple flavoring
and Sucanat; your favorite flavoring

Mix dry ingredients thoroughly. Add blended ingredients and
work with fingers until all dry ingredients are moistened and
evenly mixed. Spread on large cookie sheet or sheets. Bake at
225 degrees for 1 ½ hours or bake at lowest oven setting
overnight. Stir occasionally and bake until uniformly golden.
(Don't need to stir when baked overnight.) Cool thoroughly.
Store in airtight containers.

Yield 10 ½ cups Serves 15

Cereal Grains

Cereal grains are a great breakfast option. They are very high in fiber but low in fat. While many of us are familiar with oatmeal and grits, there are a number of other delicious grains worthy of being served for breakfast. Experiment with millet, wheat, rice, rye, and barley. Follow preparation method on the box. Try using dried fruit, (raisins, pineapple, cranberries, apricots, dates) coconut, fruit juice and even soy milk to sweeten, or Sucanat instead of the traditional white sugar.

When preparing grits, add imitation baco bits for additional flavor, instead of drowning in butter or margarine. We also like to sprinkle shredded soy cheddar cheese OR pour pimento cheese sauce over our grits.

Fruit Smoothie*

2   bananas
1 c. unsweetened crushed pineapple in its own juice
1 c. unsweetened sliced strawberries
1 c. Better Than Milk soymilk
1 t. alcohol free vanilla flavoring
½ t. alcohol free coconut flavoring
1 T honey
Ice (optional)

Blend ingredients until smooth and serve cold.

Serves 6

Delicious variations: Experiment with your favorite fruits. I have used mango, blueberry, raspberry, and fresh peaches. When fruit is in season, you don't need to additional sweetener. Try using other flavorings also. Vanilla adds sweetness.

Fruit Salad

1 can unsweetened crushed pineapple in own juice
1 can whole berry cranberry sauce/or plain cranberry sauce
(depending on your family)
2 c. frozen, unsweetened, sliced strawberries
1 c. frozen, unsweetened bluberries
1 c. frozen, unsweetened raspberries
1 c. chopped pecans

Mix all ingredients.   Allow to chill thoroughly before serving.
Excellent by the bowl, as a side dish and/or over bread.
Variation: add chopped coconut.

Serves 10

Apple Crisp

The first time Jill, our nurse made this, I tried to eat the whole
dish. This is excellent to eat along with a fruit smoothie for
breakfast.

Mix separately
2 c. fresh sliced peeled apples   2 c. rolled oats
1/4 c. diced dates   1 c. whole wheat flour
1/8 c. pineapple juice   ½ t. salt

Blend together: 1/4 c. water, 3 T. honey, 3 T. oil, 1 t. vanilla

Pour blended ingredients over dry ingredients and mix
thoroughly until dry ingredients are evenly moist. Put apple
mixture in bottom of baking pan and sprinkle topping mixture
evenly over the fruit. Bake covered with foil for 35 minutes.
Uncover and bake for an additional 10 minutes.
 Optional: Add 1/4 c. chopped nuts of your choice.
NOTE: Try out some of your favorite fruits and flavorings for
variety.

Serves 8

DINNER

Macaroni and Cheez*

2 quarts water	4 oz jar pimientos
2 c. macaroni noodles	2 T. fresh lemon juice
1 c. clean, raw cashews	2 t. salt
2 c. water	1/4 t. garlic powder
1 c. nutritional yeast flakes	1 t. onion powder

Grated soy cheese or soft bread crumbs as optional topping. I also add more garlic powder, McKay's Chicken Style Seasoning, paprika, turmeric to reach desired taste.

Bring 2 quarts water to a boil and add macaroni. Cook. While macaroni is cooking, blend cashews with 2 cups water until very smooth. Add remaining ingredients, except topping and continue blending until smooth. Drain macaroni and add to sauce. Add other suggested seasonings to taste. Stir and place in casserole dish. Bake at 350 degrees for 30 minutes. Top with optional topping and bake another 5-10 minutes.

My friend **Chaundra** uses the following for her cheese sauce. If you cannot eat nuts, it is a wonderful alternative.

2 c. water	1/4 cup pimentos
1 c. nutritional yeast flakes	1/4 cup oil (optional)
½ c. flour	2 t. salt
2 T. cornstarch	2 t. Onion flakes or power
2 T. lemon juice	1/4 t. garlic powder

Mix ingredients in a blender. Heat in sauce pan slowly. Stir until thickened. You must stir **continuously** or cheese will lump. Do not over cook or cheese will be too thick. Immediately pour over macaroni, adding your choice soy milk to thin out mixture. Add your favorite seasonings. Place in casserole dish. Sprinkle with paprika. Bake as above.

Serves 8

Chickette Pot Pie

Prepared 2-crust Pie Crust
1/3 c. clean, raw cashews
1 c. water
½ 16 oz. bag, frozen mixed vegetables
3/4 c. Worthington Chickettes, diced or torn into small pieces
2 t. plus McKay's Chicken Style Seasoning to taste
1 t. plus dried basil to taste
Garlic powder, and dried parsley to taste (optional)

Place bottom crust in pie pan. Whiz cashews and water in blender till smooth. Place in small pot and heat until it starts to thicken. Mix sauce, vegetables and seasonings in bowl. Adjust seasonings. Place in pie crust. Cover with top crust and cut slits in top. Bake in 400 degree oven until browning is noted.

Serves 6

Lasagne

6 whole grain lasagne noodles, (uncooked)
1 28-oz. jar of your favorite spaghetti sauce OR 3 ½ -4 cups of your own
½ roll of Morning Star Farm vegetarian burger crumbles
1 lb. Firm tofu
½ t. lemon juice
1/4 t. salt
½ package of Monterey Jack Soya Kass Cheese OR 1 cup of Cashew Cheese
Dried Basil, Garlic Powder, Soy Parmesan Cheese of your choice

Spray the bottom of your favorite oblong baking dish with a vegetable spray. Crumble tofu and sprinkle with lemon juice and salt. Add vegetarian burger crumbles to the spaghetti sauce. Lay three uncooked lasagne noodles in the baking dish. Pour in ½ of the meat sauce mix. Add ½ of the crumbled tofu. Sprinkle with about ½ teaspoon of basil and ½ teaspoon of garlic and some soy Parmesan cheese. Repeat the layering with remaining ingredients. Cover the top with grated soy cheese or Cashew Cheese. Sprinkle with soy Parmesan cheese. Cover and bake at 350 degrees for about 30-40 minutes. Lasagne noodles will bake up nicely.

Serves 6-8

Pasta Prima Vera

8 oz. Whole grain fettucine noodles
½ c. each sliced carrots, chopped broccoli, cauliflower, green pepper, red peppers, onions
3 cloves fresh garlic, sliced
½ c. Worthington Chickettes (optional)
1 T. olive oil

Cream Sauce

1 c. clean, raw cashews
2 c. water
½ c. Tofutti Better Than Sour Cream, optional
1 T. plus dried basil to taste
1 T. plus McKay's Chicken Style Seasoning to taste

Wash, chop and measure vegetables. Boil noodles. While noodles are boiling, mix cream sauce ingredients in blender, until smooth. Put oil in a large skillet or pot. Stir fry vegetables and optional vege-chicken. Add noodles, cream sauce and seasonings. Adjust seasonings as necessary. Sprinkle with soy Parmesan cheese.

Serves 6-8

Candied Yams

4 medium sweet potatoes
About ½ c. sweetener
> honey, pure maple syrup, Sucanat, Florida Crystals cane sugar, or brown sugar OR a combination of your favorite. Just don't use white sugar.

½ to 1 teaspoon vanilla, almond and/or maple flavoring (non-alcoholic variety)
½ t. coriander

Wash, peel and slice potatoes. Place uncooked in a baking dish and sprinkle/pour in sweetener, flavoring, and coriander. Cover and bake at 300 degrees until done. About 1 hour.

Serves 6

Honeyed Carrots*

2 pounds fresh carrots, peeled and sliced
1/4 c. honey

Place sliced carrots in sauce pan in ½ cup water. Bring to a boil and let boil for about 5 minutes, uncovered. Pour honey over carrots and cover. Turn to low and let steam till crisp tender.

Serves 8

Mashed Potatoes*

3 pounds white potatoes
½ c. Better Than Milk, soy milk
3/4 t. salt
1 t. McCormick Garlic and Herb flavored seasoning
2 t. McKay's Chicken Style Seasoning
1 t. nutritional yeast flakes
½ t. garlic powder
½ t. onion powder
Paprika and chopped parsley for garnish.

Peel and boil potatoes in small amount of water. When tender, keep about 1/4 of the boiled water in the potatoes, add other ingredients and mash. Garnish with paprika and chopped parsley.

Serves 8

Scalloped Potatoes

My husband and son always loved scalloped potatoes.
Replacing the dairy products in it was easier than I thought.
This is one of the few dishes they will eat very often.

4-medium white potatoes, washed well and sliced
1 small onion, chopped

Cream Sauce

2 c. water
1 c. clean, raw cashews
½ c. Tofutti Sour cream (optional)
2 t. plus McKay's Chicken style seasoning to taste
½ t. garlic powder
½ t. parsley (optional)

Herb flavored stuffing mix, tofu cheddar cheese OR cashew
cheese sauce

Spray oblong casserole dish with vegetable spray. Place cream
sauce ingredients in blender and blend until smooth. Adjust
seasonings to your taste. Place sliced potatoes in casserole dish.
Add chopped onion. Pour cream sauce over vegetables in dish.
Cover and bake at 350 degrees until tender. Remove from oven.
Sprinkle herb flavored bread stuffing mix and shredded soy
cheddar cheese OR cashew cheese sauce on top of the casserole.
Return to oven for about 5 minutes.

Serve 6-8

Oven Roasted Potatoes

My friend Brenda, who **claims** she is not a cook, did this recipe for her family with ease and rave reviews. Use whatever seasoning method is easiest for you.

8 red potatoes, washed well and cut up
1 medium onion, chopped
2 cloves garlic
2 T. olive oil
½ t. plus salt to taste
paprika for color (optional)

Seasoning Options
McCormick Garlic and Herb Seasoning OR
1 t. each dried basil, parsley OR
About 2 tablespoons each fresh basil, parsley and sage

Measure oil into an iron skillet. Place cut potatoes in skillet. Add your choice of seasonings and stir to coat potatoes. Roast at 400 degrees until done. Tender when pierced with fork. Stir about every 15 minutes to avoid potatoes sticking to pan. Add additional seasonings if needed.

Serves 4-6

Vegetable Rice*
2 T   olive oil
1/3 c. fresh cilantro
½ c.   shredded cabbage
1   large chopped carrot
½ c.   sweet pepper, red and green
½ c.   chopped mushrooms
1   small onion chopped
2 c.   instant brown rice
2 c.   hot water
1 T. NO MSG McKay's Chicken Style Seasoning

In large skillet (I prefer cast-iron) saute vegetables and cilantro till crisp tender. Add dry rice and stir fry for about 1 minute. Add hot water and McKay's Chicken Style seasoning. Bring to boil. Reduce heaat and let steam until rice is done, about 10-15 minutes.
Serves 8

Yellow Rice
1-14 oz. box Instant brown rice
2 t. olive oil
1 medium onion, chopped
1 lg. Bay leaf
2 t. turmeric
1 T. plus McKay's chicken style to taste
4 ½ cups hot water

Saute onions in the olive oil. While onions are sauteeing, add turmeric, McKay's Chicken Style Seasoning to hot water. Pour rice into onions and stir fry for a few minutes. Add bay leaf, and seasoned water. Bring to a boil. Cover and reduce heat. Cook until water is absorbed.
Optional: Adding about 1/4 cup each green peas, diced carrots, red/green peppers during the last few minutes of cooking make this rice very pretty.
Serves 8

Brown and Wild Rice

2 t. olive oil
1 medium onion
2 c. uncooked, long-grain brown rice
½ c. uncooked wild rice
1 T. McKays Beef Style Seasoning
6 c. hot water

Saute onions in olive oil. Add rice and stir fry for a few minutes. Add beef style seasoning and hot water. Bring mixture to a boil. Cover and reduce heat. Let simmer till done. About 45 minutes.

Optional: Add slivered almonds, sliced mushrooms and golden raisins and your favorite herbs.

Serves 8

Dirty Rice

2 c. uncooked, long-grain, brown rice
1 medium yellow onion, chopped
1 medium red onion, choped
3 cloves garlic, chopped
2 green onions, chopped
½ c. green pepper, chopped
½ c. red pepper, chopped
1 T. olive oil
1 t. McKay's Chicken Style Seasoning
3 T. plus dried basil to taste
1 T. dried parsley
½ c. Worthington Chickettes, torn pieces
½ c. vegetarian turkey, chopped
½ c. vegetarian beef crumbles
½ c. vegetarian ham, chopped
½ c. vegetarian pepperoni, optional
Bragg's Liquid Aminoes, optional

Cook rice. In a separate pan, saute vegetables in olive oil. Add chopped veggie meat, and seasonings. Add cooked rice and stir thoroughly. Add additional McKay's Chicken Style seasoning, Bragg's Liquid Aminoes, to taste. If the rice is not "dirty" enough, add paprika.

Variations:
Use your favorite vegetables, broccoli, cauliflower, carrots, etc. instead of vegetarian meats.
Wonderful Jamacian variation, given to me by Jennifer Bent. Saute Vegetarian Tuno with vegetables, omitting other vegetarian meats. Add cooked rice and mix thoroughly.

Serves 8

Jamaican Rice and Peas

I learned to cook this recipe while in college. So many of my friends were from the Caribbean islands. My friend Elsie showed me how to master it. When I decided to eat brown rice, I couldn't quite get this dish done without it looking like oatmeal. Thank God for instant brown rice. My son tries to eat the whole pot.

1-15 oz. can kidney beans-light red, dark red or small red
1-14 oz. can coconut milk
1-14 oz. box instant brown rice
2 cloves garlic, chopped
2 green onions, chopped
salt to taste
sprig of fresh thyme
Water to bring bean juice liquid, and coconut milk amount to 4 3/4 cups

Drain bean liquid into a measuring cup. Add coconut milk and enough water to measure 4 3/4 cups. Place liquid, beans, onions, garlic and thyme in a large pot. Add salt to taste. Let boil gently for about 10 minutes. Add rice, stir and bring to rapid boil. Cover and reduce heat. Simmer until water is absorbed. Enjoy mon!☺

Serves 8

Haystacks - A One-Dish Meal

Your Choice Vegetarian Chili - homemade or canned
1 (7-ounce) bag regular-size corn chips
1 medium head dark green lettuce, shredded
3 large tomatoes, diced
2 cups shredded, soy cheddar or Monterey jack cheese
Vinegar free taco sauce
Optional: Olives, chopped onion, Tofutti Better than Sour
Cream, sliced avocado or guacamole.

Prepare chili; keep warm. On dinner plates layer 1 cup corn
chips, 3/4 cup shredded lettuce, 1 cup chili, 1/3 cup shredded
cheese, ½ cup diced tomato. Top with taco sauce and optional
items, if desired. Serve immediately.

Serves 6-8

**This is an excellent, quick, satisfying meal, that is
high in protein and fiber.**

Callaloo*

While visiting my parents when they lived in Florida, my mom
served this dish. She used spinach. When I got home, I got the
callaloo and boy did it go over real well. My Jamaican friend
Jennifer Bent (who was one of our meat-eating patients who
converted herself and her husband), serves this to her meat-
eating friends and family. They love it!!!!! (Most of the
Jamaican recipes included with this collection are with
Jennifer's suggestion)

1   medium onion, chopped
2   cloves garlic, chopped
1   T Olive oil
3   pounds Spinach (fresh) or Callaloo, chopped
1/4 - ½   cup water
1/4 c. coconut milk
2   teaspoons McKay's NO MSG Chicken Style Seasoning
1/4 cup Worthington TUNO
1   small tomato, chopped

Wash the spinach or callaloo thoroughly. Cut off lower ends of
stems. Chop or cut into strips. In skillet saute onions and garlic
in olive oil. Add chopped spinach, water, coconut milk, and
seasonings. Cover and steam till almost tender (about 6-8
minutes). Add tuno and chopped tomato and steam another few
minutes.

Serves 6

Callaloo & Okra

3 pounds callaloo, chopped
5-6 okra, chopped
1 medium onion, chopped
1 medium tomato, diced
1 small green pepper, chopped
1 small red pepper, chopped
1 t. oil

Steam callaloo and okra in a small amount of water until done.
While steaming, saute vegetables in a small amount of oil.
Combine both mixtures, cover and let simmer about 10-15
minutes.

Serves 6

Collard Greens

2 pounds collard greens
3 T. olive oil
1 medium red onion, finely chopped
2 gloves garlic, crushed
1 red bell pepper, seeded, sliced
2/3 c. vegetable broth or water
1 T. plus McKay's Chicken Style Seasoning to taste
Bakon Seasoning or Imitation Baco Bits to taste

Wash collard greens in several changes of water. Strip leaves
from stalks. On cutting board, pile leaves in stacks and slice
very thinly Steam over pan of boiling water until slightly wilted,
about 5 minutes. Place greens in strainer or colander and press
out excess water. Transfer to large plate and set aside to cool.
In large saucepan, heat the oil; saute the onions until browned.
Add garlic and stir fry 1-2 minutes. Add greens, bell pepper and
remaining broth. Mix well. Over low heat , cover and cook 15
minutes or until of desired tenderness.

Serves 6-8

Turnip Greens and Cabbage

I had cooked some turnips that were very bitter. Knowing my son would not want them, I decided to add some chopped cabbage. The cabbage sweetened those turnips right up. It was a hit! This is my favorite way to eat turnips now. Sometimes I will combine turnips, mustard and kale and cook this way too.

2 bunches turnip greens
1 small head green cabbage, chopped
1 medium onion, chopped
2 cloves garlic, chopped
1 T. olive oil
1 T. plus McKay's Chicken Style seasoning to taste
2/3 c. vegetable broth or water

Wash turnip greens in several changes of water. On cutting board, pile leaves in stacks and slice. Steam over pan of boiling water until slightly wilted, about 5 minutes. Place greens in strainer or colander and press out excess water. Transfer to large plate and set aside to cool. In large saucepan, heat the oil; saute the onions until browned. Add garlic and stir fry 1-2 minutes. Add greens and broth you steamed the greens over. Add seasonings and mix well. Cook about 15 minutes. Add chopped cabbage and steam till cabbage is done. Serve with black eyed peas, and cornbread. Umm, umm, good!!!

Serves 6-8

Steamed Cabbage

My brother Steve comes for dinner if he knows we're having **Debbie's** cabbage. This is really good.

1 medium head cabbage, chopped (use all leaves, including green outer leaves)
1 medium onion, sliced into strips
1 T. plus McKay's Chicken Style to taste
2 t. olive oil
½ c. water (add more if needed)
BAKON to taste (optional)

Pour water in medium pot and bring to boil. Add cabbage, onion, and seasonings. Bring to boil again. Stir, cover and reduce heat. Simmer till done. (I prefer crisp tender.) Add olive oil and optional BAKON to taste. Try not to eat it all at one setting.

Option: add sweet peppers, fresh garlic, dill.
Serves 6-8

Succotash

½ c. water
1 16 oz. bag, frozen lima beans
1 16 oz. bag frozen corn
1 2 ½ oz jar chopped pimento OR ½ cup chopped sweet red pepper
1 T. imitation Baco Bits
2 t. plus McKay's Chicken Style seasoning to taste
½ t. olive oil (optional)

Pour water into saucepan and bring to a boil. Add lima beans. Bring to another boil, reduce heat and simmer until almost done, about 20 minutes. Add corn, and pimento/pepper, and seasonings. Bring to boil again. Reduce and simmer for another 5-7 minutes. Add optional olive oil and serve.
Serves 6-8

Festive Corn

½ c. water
1 16 oz. bag frozen corn
1 2 ½ oz. jar chopped pimento OR ½ cup chopped sweet red pepper
1/4 t. cumin
dash salt

Pour water into saucepan and bring to a boil. Add corn. Bring to another boil, reduce heat and simmer until done. Add seasonings and pimento/pepper. Stir and serve.
Serves 6-8

Southern Style Fried Corn

It's kind of hard to make fried corn without meat drippings and milk. But, it's not impossible. I created this recipe while talking to my friend Joann on the phone. As I was tasting and adjusting the seasonings, she could tell I was gettin' it right, and warned me not to eat it up myself. When I served it, my momma and her girlfriend Alfreda, tried to eat it all up.

4 ears fresh corn, yellow and/or white
2 t. olive oil
1 slice Yves Canadian Bacon, chopped
4 slices Yves Pepperoni, chopped
1 T. imitation baco bits
1 c. plus additional soy milk, as needed
salt and sugar to taste

Wash corn and cut off cob. Heat oil in cast iron skillet. Add vegetarian meats and heat. (This seasons the oil.) Add corn and one cup of soy milk. Add sugar and salt. Bring to boil. Reduce heat and simmer until done. Add milk if necessary as mixture thickens.

Serves 6

Vanessa's Summer Squash

I have tried for 15 years to get my husband to eat squash without a fight. Our friend, Vanessa prepared this dish at her house for an after church dinner. When Eddie asked me if I enjoyed the squash that she made, I nearly fainted. Thanks Vanessa!!

1 medium onion, sliced
4 medium summer squash, green and yellow, or all one color
1 T. dried basil
2-3 T. McKay's Chicken Style Seasoning
½ - 1 t. garlic powder
1 - 2 T. oil

Slice onion and separate into rings. Saute in olive oil. Add sliced squash and seasonings. Cover and simmer until tender. Will make its own broth. Enjoy!

Serves 4-6

ENTREES

What about meat? When you have eaten flesh most of your life, your plate suddenly seems empty if all you see is vegetables. Fortunately, there are some delicious 'meat substitutes' that can be used instead. Some of them you can make yourself. Others are available commercially. Following are some that my family seems to love. Ideas for cooking beans, a wonderful source of plant protein, are also included.

Oat Burgers

2 c. dry oats	1 t. dried basil
1 medium onion, chopped fine	½ t. salt
1 c. walnuts, ground	1 t. McKay's Chicken Style
3/4 cup soy milk	2-3 T. Nutritional Yeast Flakes
1/4 cup Braggs Liquid Aminoes	1 T. gluten Flour
1 t. sage	½ c. bread crumbs
1 large garlic clove, minced	1 t. olive oil (optional)

Place oats, onion, garlic and walnuts in a mixing bowl. Heat milk and Braggs Liquid Aminoes. Add seasonings to heated liquid. Pour liquid mixture into dry ingredients. Let stand about 5-10 minutes. Mixture should be slightly stiff. If not, add some more bread crumbs. Form into patties and place on a baking sheet that has been sprayed with vegetable spray. Bake at 350 degrees until browned. Turn once during baking. Delicious when served with gravy and mashed potatoes. Also good on burger bun with lettuce and tomato and onion.

Millet Burgers

When I was away at Wildwood, Stephanie was one of many
church members who made sure my family was fed. Here is my
version of some burgers she made. They are good dry. But of
course gravy always adds a little something.

2 c. cooked millet (½ cup millet in 2 c. water)
1 t. garlic powder
2 T. gluten flour
1 large onion, chopped
1/4 c. chopped walnuts
1 cup tofu, crumbled
3 T. Braggs Liquid Amino
½ cup plain bread crumbs
1 T. nutritional yeast flakes
2 t. plus McKay's Chicken Style Seasoning to taste
1 t. dried basil
dash of oregano and sage
1 t. olive oil (optional)
Cook millet (takes 30-45 minutes). Let cool and mix with all
other ingredients. Form into patties and place in baking dish
that has been sprayed with a vegetable spray. Bake at 350
degrees until golden brown. Turn once.

Quick Vegetarian Chili

1 16 oz. can chili beans
1 16 oz. can pink beans
1 16 oz. can kidney beans
½ roll Morningstar Farms Burger Crumbles
1 15 oz. can, plain tomato sauce
1 t. garlic powder
2 t. cumin
1/4 - 1/3 cup Vinegar-free Salsa
Pour all ingredients into a large pot. Heat until bubbly. Adjust
to your taste if necessary.   Serve in a bowl, in haystacks or over
rice.
Serves 6-8

Jamaican Patty

1 recipe pie crust dough, Jamaican variation
½ c. each of the following

> Veggie ground round OR Your favorite Vegetarian beef substitute
> onion, chopped
> sweet red pepper, chopped
> sweet green pepper, chopped
> frozen green peas

Optional seasonings: garlic powder, sage, thyme, McKay's Beef Style Seasoning

Saute vegetarian meat and vegetables in oil or non-stick skillet sprayed with vegetable spray. Add optional seasonings. Let mixture cool. While cooling, roll dough out onto floured area. Cut into circles or squares. Place about 1 heaping tablespoon of filling into each pastry piece. Fold in half and seal with water or a fork. Place on baking sheet and bake at 400 degrees until golden brown 12-15 minutes.

Variation: Use chopped vegetables (carrots, peas, potatoes) instead for filling.

Ackee and Tuno

1 roll Worthington Tuno
1 14 oz can Ackee OR 1 pound firm tofu diced and sprinkled with turmeric (for ackee color)
1 medium onion, chopped
1 large tomato, chopped
1 medium green pepper, chopped

Saute vegetables. Add tuno and ackee. Simmer for about 15 minutes. Serve.

Serves 4-6

Cooking Beans

Many people don't cook beans because of the time it takes and the gas that results from eating them. They are, however, a wonderful source of fiber, protein and other phytochemicals. I surely do eat my share. When cooking them, if you soak them first, then pour off the water before cooking them, they are not as gassy. I cook mine exclusively in a crock pot and don't seem to have the gas problem either. Instead if giving you bean recipes, here are some tips. I have found that less seasoning for beans is best. When you let the beans cook up first without too much seasoning in them, you really get their full taste. Add suggested seasonings to taste. Add salt and 1-2 teaspoons oil at the end of cooking time. Serve over rice, or in a bowl with cornbread.

BEAN COOKING TIPS	
To **any** 1 pound of beans I cook I always add	1 medium onion 2 cloves garlic
To Pinto Beans, also add suggested amount plus more to taste	2 t. Cumin 1 T. McKay's Chicken Style
To Black-eyed Peas, also add suggested amount, plus more to taste	1 T. McKay's Chicken Style 2 t. BAKON 2 t. Basil
To Black Beans, also add suggested amount, plus more to taste	1 T. Cumin 1 T. McKay's Chicken Style 1 medium diced tomato
To Northern Beans, also add suggested amount, plus more to taste	2 t. McKay's Chicken Style 1 t. BAKON 1 t. Parsley 1 T. imitation baco bits
To Lentils also add 1 medium white potato, diced 1 large carrot, diced ½ medium sweet red pepper, chopped and suggested seasoning amount, plus more to taste	2 t. McKay's Chicken Style 1 t. BAKON 1 t. Basil ½ t. cumin (optional)

Baked Chickettes

Chickette roll - by Worthington Foods
Garlic Herb Salad Dressing, made with tofu
Corn Flake Crumbs seasoned with chicken seasoning, garlic, paprika

Thaw chickette roll. Tear chickette into serving pieces. Dip in salad dressing and dredge in cornflake crumbs. Place in single layer in a baking dish that has been sprayed with vegetable spray or lightly oiled. Bake in 400 degree oven until browned. Turn halfway through cooking.

Barbeque Chickettes

While I avoid FRYING, this recipe is for those who really, really need the taste and haven't quite decided to bake everything. I eat this occasionally, ONLY!!!

1 roll Worthington Chickettes
1 recipe Donna's Momma's Barbeque Sauce

Thaw roll of chickettes. Tear into serving size pieces. Fry in canola oil until golden brown and crisp. Place in dish and pour barbecue sauce over. Try not to eat it all up yourself!

Ivey's New Favorite Pizza

This is my son's most favorite meal to prepare. Because we used to live at a local pizzeria☺, we had to do something to help us make the adjustment. We have found one commercial soy cheese that was perfect. If you want to ALWAYS avoid dairy (most soy cheeses contain caseinate, a milk protein), then use the Cashew Cheese Sauce instead.

Pizza crust - homemade, store bought, pita bread, bagel, burger bun

Sauce - homemade, store bought or spaghetti sauce

Toppings - cheese, onions, mushrooms, black olives, veggie burger, veggie pepperoni, soy Parmesan cheese

Place crust in oven proof dish. Spoon on sauce. Sprinkle on toppings. Bake at 450 till done.

BREADS

YEAST CORNBREAD

2 cups warm water
2 T. dry yeast
4 T. honey
4 T. raw sugar
2 t. salt
1/3 c. oil

2 1/4 c. cornmeal
3/4 c. unbleached all purpose flour
1/4 c. whole wheat pastry flour
1/4 c. soy flour

Mix first four ingredients together and let set until bubbly (5-10 minutes). Combine remaining ingredients and mix well. Pour into 9" x 12" baking dish that has been sprayed. Let rise for 20-30 minutes. Bake at 350 degrees for 30-45 minutes.

Serves 8

QUICK CORNBREAD

2 c. whole grain cornmeal
4 t. baking powder
1 t. salt
2 EnerG egg replacers
1 T. wheat germ

2 T. sweetener (optional)
1 ½ c. soy milk
4 T. Willow Run Margarine
Hot water

Heat oven to 400 degrees. Place margarine in iron skillet and put in oven to melt. Mix all dry ingredients. Add melted margarine and soy milk to dry ingredients. Mix well. Add just enough hot water to make a smooth batter. Place in skillet and bake at 400 degrees until done.

Delicious Variation
Replace margarine with 2 T. oil and 1 heaping T. Tofutti Better Than Sour Cream. Use honey as the sweetener.

Serves 8

Cornbread Dressing

1 recipe your favorite cornbread
1 medium onion, chopped
1 stalk celery, chopped
½ medium green pepper
2 c. herb flavored, cubed stuffing mix
2 c. hot water
2 T. plus McKays Chicken Style to taste
1 t. garlic powder

Saute onion, celery and peppers in a little olive oil. Crumble cornbread and add to it dry, seasoned stuffing mix, and sauteed vegetables. Add garlic powder, sage, and McKays Chicken Style to water. Pour into dried mixture to desired moistness. (Asparagus juice gives a WONDERFUL turkey flavor, and I sometimes add small, torn pieces of Worthington Chickettes to it also.)

Pour mixture in baking dish that has been sprayed with vegetable spray. Bake covered (if you like it soft) or uncovered (if you like it drier), at 350 degrees until done. About 30-45 minutes.

Serves 6-8

SOUPS

Chickette Noodle Soup

6 c. water
1 ½ cup flat noodles
½ c. green peas
1 large carrot, diced
½ c. Worthington Chickettes, torn into small pieces
1 T. plus McKay's Chicken Style Seasoning to taste
½ t. plus garlic powder to taste
1 t. parsley (optional)
1 T. cornstarch
½ c. water

Pour water into large pot and bring to a boil. Add noodles and
cook. When nearly done add peas, carrots, chickettes and
seasonings. Dissolve cornstarch in additional ½ cup water and
add to soup. Let bubble for about 10 minutes, adding more
water if necessary. Serve.

Variation: add broccoli instead of OR in addition to peas

Serves 4-6

Creamy Potato Soup

7 cups water
4 medium potatoes, peeled and diced
1 medium onion, chopped
2 cloves garlic, chopped
1 c. water
½ c. clean, raw cashews
1 T. plus McKay's Chicken Style Seasoning to taste
1 T. Imitation baco bits
1 t. parsley
½ t. basil (optional)

Garnish: Dash of paprika and grated soy cheese

Pour water, potatoes, onions, and garlic in a large pot. Bring to a boil and cook till tender. While vegetables are boiling, blend 1 cup water and cashews in blender. When vegetables are done, add cashew mixture, and seasonings. Adjust to taste. Slowly add more water if too thick. Let simmer about 15 minutes. Add garnish and serve.

Serves 4-6

SALADS/DRESSINGS/SAUCES

TOSSED SALAD
4 cups lettuce - Green Leaf, Romaine, Curly Lettuce (no iceberg) shredded
1 Medium Diced Tomato
½ Medium Red Onion, sliced and separated into rings
½ c. yellow and green squash
1 large carrot, grated
3/4 c. red, green, yellow peppers, julienned
½ c. cucumbers, thinly sliced
3/4 c. broccoli and cauliflower, flowerets
½ c. red cabbage, shredded
Optional toppings: **If you like**, raisins, peanuts, your choice of beans, corn, peas, imitation baco bits, sesame seed, flax seed, black olives, ripe green olives, kidney or garbanzo beans, kernel corn, green cabbage, peanuts, croutons.

Layer or toss in your favorite salad bowl.

Yield 6 servings

Caesar Salad
I used to love to eat Caesar Salad. Well, I didn't know that there were anchovies in it. Here is my healthier variation.

6 c. Romaine lettuce, torn into bite-size pieces
3 c. green leaf lettuce or spinach leaves, torn into bite-size pieces
2 carrots, peeled and grated
½ c. black olives (optional)
2 c. croutons
Caesar-Salad dressing

Combine lettuce, carrots, 1 ½ cups of the croutons. Drizzle dressing over salad mixture. Toss well to coat evenly. Top with remaining ½ cup croutons. Soy Parmesan cheese can be sprinkled on as a topping.

Caesar Salad Dressing

1 pkg. Soft silken tofu   2 t. plus honey to taste
3 T. vegetable oil   3/4 t. salt
1 ½ T. lemon juice
Combine ingredients and blend until smooth.

ADD:*2-3 tablespoons water, 1-2 teaspoons fresh lemon juice, 1-2 garlic cloves, minced, 2 T. dried basil, 2 t. dried parsley, 1/4 t. dill, dash oregano.

Combine in blender or food processor; process well. Set dressing aside. Dressing should be thin. If needed, add additional water to thin the dressing. Garlic cloves make it spicy!

TOFU MAYONNAISE

These delicious mayonnaise alternatives can be used whenever mayonnaise is called for. Vary by adding herbs such as dill, basil, or rosemary for a delicious salad dressing or dip. Firm tofu will produce a thicker more dip-like consistency. Be sure to use within 7-10 days.

Tofu Mayonnaise* - 1

1 lb. soft, crumbled tofu	1 t. garlic powder
½ c. water	½ c canola oil
1 t. salt	1/4-1/2 c. fresh lemon juice
2 ½ t. onion powder	1/4 c. honey (optional)

Nutritional yeast flakes, bakon seasoning, turmeric to taste
Rinse, drain, crumble and measure tofu. Put into blender and add remaining ingredients. Blend on high for one minute until creamy. Keep refrigerated.

Tofu Mayonnaise - 2

1 package soft or firm silken tofu	1 ½ T. honey
2 T. plus 2 t. lemon juice	3/4 t. salt
6 T. oil	

In blender or food processor, combine all ingredients and process for one minute or until smooth. Refrigerate until serving time.

Tartar Sauce

1 c. tofu mayonnaise
½ c. PA's Pickle Relish
2 heaping T. chopped onion
Garlic powder, turmeric to taste

Mix all ingredients. Let chill. Serve with Salmonette Patties.

Variation: I sometimes add an additional 1/4 c. soy sour cream.

Eddie's French Salad Dressing*

1 c.	soy, corn, safflower or canola oil
1/3 c	fresh lemon juice
1/3 c.	honey
½ T.	paprika
1-10 oz.	can tomato puree
½ T.	onion powder
1 t.	garlic powder
1 t.	salt

Blend all ingredients on high for 30 seconds. Chill in covered container.
Yield: 2 ½ cups

Pammie's Easy Tofu Salad Dressing

Right after my diagnosis, my friend Pam Byoune came over for dinner. We discussed how we could have a creamy salad dressing without using dairy. As we talked, we decided to do the following recipe. We nearly licked the blender clean!!

1 Packet of Garlic Herb, Zesty Italian or Zesty Herb Good Seasons Salad Dressing Mix
1/4 c. fresh lemon juice
2 T.- ½ c. water depending on how thick/thin you want dressing to be
1/4 - ½ c. canola oil
1/4 package or more of silken, soft tofu

Blend all ingredients in blender. Pour into container and chill till ready to serve

Chikin/Tuno Salad

2 c. your favorite pasta
½ roll Worthington Tuno
½ can Worthington Fri-Chik
1 t. plus basil to taste
½ t. plus garlic powder to taste

1/3 c. frozen green peas
1 medium carrot, shredded
2 t. McKay's Chicken Style
½ recipe soy mayonnaise
salt to taste (optional)

Boil pasta. Rinse and drain. Grate Fri-Chik into pasta. Add other ingredients and stir. Adjust seasonings. If too dry, add some of the Fri-Chik juice.

Variation: Mix vegetarian meats with mayonnaise, onions and your favorite seasonings to make a delicious
"Tuno" salad for sandwiches.

Serves 6-8

Potato Salad

5 lbs. Potatoes, boiled and diced
1 recipe soy mayonnaise
1 c. chopped vegetables
(your choice of carrots, red/green pepper, red onion, green/black olives)
½ c. PA's Pickle Relish, made with lemon juice instead of vinegar
Season to taste with garlic powder, turmeric, salt, paprika, McKay's Chicken Style Seasoning

Mix all vegetables. Add seasonings SLOWLY to taste.

OPTIONAL: Fold in **gently**, 2 T. crumbled tofu seasoned with turmeric and garlic (looks like egg yolk)

Serves 6-8

Donna Momma's Barbecue Sauce

So much of the commercial sauces have ingredients that are really harmful to the digestive system. I gave up those that had vinegar in them and really needed some kind of replacement. My mom and I worked on a barbecue sauce. One day, Connie Flint, of WAOK radio commented on how good "Donna Momma's Barbecue" was-thus the name. When I make it, I refrigerate what I don't use right away. My family loves it.

1 - 28 oz. can tomato puree
1 - 28 oz. can tomato sauce
1 large onion, chopped
2-3 lg. garlic cloves, chopped
1/4 c. canola oil
½ c. Sucanat
2 T. molasses
1 t. turmeric

1 t. salt
2 T. dried parsley
1/4 t. crushed red pepper (opt.)
2 T. honey
2 T. Bragg's Liquid Aminoes
½ c. fresh lemon juice
1-20 oz. jar peach preserves
1-2 T. Wrights's liquid smoke

In large sauce pan (I use a cast-iron skillet), saute onions and garlic in oil. Add all other ingredients except lemon juice, peach preserves and liquid smoke. Cover and let simmer about 20 minutes. Add lemon juice, peach preserves and liquid smoke. Let simmer another 15 - 20 minutes till flavors blend. Serve as you would any commercial barbecue sauce. Makes especially good Barbecue Chickettes.

Nacho Cheese Dip

2 C. water
1/4 C. clean, raw cashews
4 oz. jar pimientos
½ - 1 c. nutritional yeast flakes (secret for cheezy taste)
1 ½ -2 T. cornstarch or arrowroot
1 T. fresh lemon juice (optional)
1 ½ T. salt
½ T. onion flakes or powder
1/4 T. garlic powder
½ T. cumin, heaping

Blend cashews in about ½ cup of the water until very smooth.
Add remaining water and other ingredients and continue
blending until smooth. Simmer in a heavy saucepan until
thickened, Stirring constantly(5-6 Minutes). Serve as dip or pour
over vegetables.

Option: Add vegetarian burger, black olives, vinegar-free salsa.
We made this for the annual winter sports gathering and
the men absolutely loved it!!!!!!!!!!!!
Omit cumin and eat as a plain cheez sauce

DESSERTS

Whole Grain Pie Crust

2/3 c. unbleached all purpose flour	1 t. salt
2/3 c. oat flour	½ cup water
2/3 c. whole wheat pastry flour	½ cup oil

In a bowl, mix flour and salt. In a separate bowl mix water and oil together with a wire whip. Add liquid to dry ingredients. Form into ball. Cut ball in half. Place one piece between two pieces of waxed paper, roll out dough into pie shape. Remove top sheet of waxed paper and place pie crust into pie pan. Remove other piece of waxed paper. Do the same to the other piece of dough. Fill with desired topping.

Yield: 2 pie crusts

Delicious Variations:
For **savory crust** used in pot pies add 1 t. basil
For **Caribbean Patty** crust add ½ - 3/4 t. turmeric
For **fruit cobbler crust** use
       1 1/4 cup unbleached all purpose flour and 3/4 cup
whole   wheat pastry flour
       After putting top crust on cobbler, brush lightly with
       water and sprinkle on evaporated cane juice sugar

Fruit Cobbler

My husband Eddie loves cobbler. I have never really been impressed with it. All the ones I had ever eaten had too much doughy crust. When I finally tried this recipe, it was a hit. The blueberry variation is even more tasty to me. (and full of cancer fighting phytochemicals) I think I'm hooked. I eat it for breakfast. If you serve it with soy vanilla ice cream, you might get slapped!!!

Prepared pastry crust for 2 crust pie

2-29 oz cans peaches, in own juice **OR** 4 cups fresh or frozen peaches
½ cup Sucanat
1/4 - ½ cup plain flour
1 t. vanilla plus more to taste
1 t. coriander
dash of salt

Prepare crust. Place 2/3 of the pie crust dough, in your favorite 8 x 8 baking dish. Save remaining 1/3 for top. Drain fruit. Mix with all other ingredients. Taste and adjust if necessary. Pour into pie crust. Cover with remaining dough. Pinch edges closed. Cut decorative slits in the top of crust. Bake in 350 degree oven until browning is noted - about 40 minutes.

Variation: Use 4 cups fresh or frozen blueberries and evaporated cane juice crystals instead of Sucanat. Cut top crust in strips and lattice across the top of the cobbler.

Potato Pie

My friend Al is a Southern man who **knows** how to cook potato pie. The traditional one is loaded with butter, milk and eggs. Here is his version of potato pie. It is absolutely delicious.

6 medium sweet potatoes, cooked and mashed
1/4 c. flour
1 ½ c. evaporated cane juice sugar
½ c. soy margarine, melted
1 t. lemon extract
pinch of salt

Mix all ingredients well. Pour into prepared pie pan. This recipe usually makes three regular pies or two deep dish pies. Bake at 375 till browning is noted, about 40 minutes.

Variation: I substitute Sucanat for the evaporated cane juice, add soy milk for creaminess, and about ½ - 1 t. coriander. The final product is browner and has a richer, more pungent taste. It reminded me of pies my Auntie Sarah and Great-Grandma Lula used to bake.

Tofu Cheesecake
BLEND

1 lb. firm or medium firm tofu	½ t. salt
½ c. canola oil	1 T. vanilla
3/4 c. honey	
3 ½ T. fresh lemon juice	

Pour blended ingredients into prepared graham cracker pie crust and bake at 350 degrees for 30 minutes, then reduce oven to 250 degrees and bake for 20-30 minutes till inserted toothpick comes out clean. Chill and cover with fruit sauce - blueberry, cherry, pineapple.

Delicious Variation
> Add ½ t. almond or orange extract
> Add 1 teaspoon each coconut and pineapple flavoring.
> Add 1 container Tofutti Better Than Cream Cheese
> When cheesecake is through baking, let cool to room temperature then top with 1 8 oz. can drained, crushed pineapple and garnish with shredded coconut.
> Garnish with carob chips and slivered almonds

Fruit Sauce
1-12 oz can frozen apple juice, or white grape juice
2-3 t. cornstarch
1 - 2 c. your favorite fresh fruit, strawberries, blueberries, etc.

Pour fruit juice and cornstarch into small pot. Heat until thickened, stirring constantly. Remove from heat and let cool. Add fruit and stir. Use as a topping for cheesecakes, pancakes, waffles.

NOTE: One can of frozen apple juice concentrate, cornstarch and coriander to taste makes a wonderful, fruit-juice sweetened **apple pie.** Use it in your favorite recipe in place of refined white sugar..

Pineapple Cheesecake

This recipe is delicious, contains NO dairy, and is from the *Silver Hills Guest House Cookbook*.

2 T. Emes unflavoured vegetable gelatin
3/4 c. pineapple juice
1 c. boiling pineapple juice
1/3 c. honey
1 c. raw cashews
1/4 c. chopped coconut
½ t. salt
6 ice cubes
1-10 oz. Can crushed pineapple, drained

Place gelatin and 3/4 cup pineapple juice in a blender and let soak for 10 minutes. Pour 1 cup boiling pineapple juice over the soaked mixture and blend briefly to dissolve gelatin. Add honey, cashews, coconut and salt to blender and blend until creamy. Add ice cubes to the blender until the mixture reaches the 1 quart mark. Blend until smooth. Pour blended mixture into a bowl and gently fold in crushed pineapple. Pour over your favorite baked crumb crust or into parfait glasses. Let stand until set and serve with a fruit topping. (Use other fruit juice concentrates to vary the cheesecake flavor. Strawberry was a hit!)

Fudgy Carob Brownies

1 c. whole wheat pastry flour
1 c. oat flour   2/3 c. soy milk
1 c. coarsely chopped walnuts   1 tsp. salt
½ c. oil   1 ½ tsp. coffee substitute
1 c. honey   ½ c. carob powder
4 tsp. vanilla

Before making brownies, preheat oven to 375 degrees and spray
an 8x8 baking dish. In bowl stir together first three ingredients.
Blend remaining ingredients on high for one minute. Pour into
dry ingredients and fold together quickly. Spread batter into
baking dish and bake at 375 degrees for 15 minutes. Reduce
heat to 350 degrees and bake 15 minutes more. Do not
overbake. Cool, cut into squares. May frost. I sometimes add
about 3/4 cup carob chips to batter. DEELISH!!!!

Serves 6-8

Carob Candy

1 c. Carob Chips
1 c. peanut butter
½ -1 c. chopped nuts

Place carob chips, peanut butter, and nuts in a microwave safe
bowl. Microwave (or melt in a double broiler) until chips are
softened/melted. Stir and pour batter into a lightly oiled pan.
Chill. Cut into squares and serve.
Delicious variations:
          Add ½ -1 cup granola
          Add ½ - 1 cup pure maple syrup
          Add chopped coconut
Serving suggestion: place in mini cupcake cups and chill.
(Looks like Reese's)

Vegan Hummingbird Cake

I first tasted hummingbird cake at my friend Joan's house when I lived in Athens, GA. We loved it, and I made it often. After changing my diet I wanted a substitute. When my friend Jill (who is vegan) makes it for her family, she sometimes cuts back on the oil and sugar and makes into bread or muffins. I hesitated including it in the book but, my friend Debbie insisted. **I do not eat this often!!!!!!!** But it's a dessert idea when you just must have something sweet. Here's what I've come up with.

2 c. plain, unbleached flour
1 c. whole wheat pastry flour
1 c. Florida Crystals
1 c. Sucanat
1 t. salt
2 t. baking powder
1 c. canola oil
3 Ener-G Egg Replacesr
6 T. soy milk
1-8 oz. can, crushed pineapple, with juice
3 medium, ripe bananas, mashed
1 cup chopped nuts, your choice (optional)
2 t. vanilla
1 t. coriander

Sift dry ingredients into bowl. Add liquid ingredients and stir till mixed thoroughly. Pour into prepared cake pan--bundt or 2-9" layer pans. Bake at 350 till done. Cake will pull away from edge of pan. Test center with toothpick. Let cool and ice with one of the following.

Tofu Cream Cheese Frosting

Mix ½ pound tofu cream cheese, 2 T. honey and ½ t. vanilla extract. Spread on cake. Garnish with chopped nuts. Double recipe if making a layer cake.

Pineapple/Cream Cheese Frosting

1-6 oz. can pineapple juice
1-3 t. cornstarch
1/4 c. brown sugar
1/4 c. Florida Crystals
1 t. pineapple extract
½ container Tofutti Better Than Cream Cheese

In small saucepan, mix all ingredients. (I like to whisk them together). Place over medium heat. Heat until thickened, stirring constantly to avoid lumping. Let cool and spread on cake. Garnish with chopped nuts.

Auntie Donna's Yum Yum Ice Cream*
2 c. water
1 c. Better Than Milk soy milk powder, plain
1 pkg. firm, silken tofu
1 c. sweetener
½-3/4 pkg. Tofutti Better Than Cream Cheese
2 T. powdered Egg Replacer, optional
2 t. alcohol-free vanilla flavoring
Optional: 3/4 cup your choice fruit. Strawberry is our favorite.

Place all ingredients in blender and blend until smooth. Place in ice cream freezer and follow manufacturer's directions. Makes about 1 quart.
Note: Sweetener can be 1 cup of evaporated cane juice **OR** honey **OR** fruit juice concentrate **OR** Sucanat **OR** maple syrup **OR** any combination of the above.
Use YOUR favorite soy milk instead of Better Than Milk
Variations:
Carob Flavor - Add ½ cup carob powder' sweeten with 1/3 cup honey, 1/3 cup Sucanat and 1/3 cup maple syrup. Add mint flavor too!!

Butter Pecan - Add 2 teaspoons alcohol-free butter flavoring. Add ½ - 3/4 cup chopped pecans during last 5 minutes of freezing.

Maple Walnut/Carob Chip - Add 2 teaspoons alcohol-free maple flavoring. Add ½ cup chopped walnuts and ½ cup carob chips during last 5 minutes of freezing process.

Reese's Peanut Butter Cup - Add broken pieces of Carob Candy during the last five minutes of freezing process.

Koffee - Add 2 Heaping T. of Roma to blender mix.

Pecan/Carob Chip - Add ½ cup nuts and ½ cup carob chips during last 5 minutes of freezing process.

Old Fashioned Carob Chip Cookies

This is a variation of a recipe I found in *Natural Health* magazine. My friend Pam does not toast or grind her grains, and they are still delicious.

1 ½ c. old-fashioned rolled oats, toasted and ground to a coarse meal in a food processor
1   c. whole wheat pastry flour
½   t. salt
½   t. baking powder
1   c. whole raw almonds, toasted and chopped
1   c. carob chips
½   c. canola oil
½   c. maple syrup
2   t. vanilla extract

1. Position rack in middle of oven and preheat oven to 375 degrees.
2. Place ground oats, flour, salt and baking powder in large bowl. Stir well with wire whisk. Add nuts and chips and stir again.
3. Combine oil, syrup and vanilla in small bowl. Whisk vigorously until emulsified. Stir wet ingredients into dry just until oat mixture is absorbed. If dough seems too sticky to handle, refrigerate 15 minutes or so and then proceed.
4. Drop rounded tablespoons of dough onto prepared baking sheets about ½ inches apart. Flatten dough with fingers to a thickness of 1/3 inch and smooth edges.
5. Slide one sheet into oven and bake until cookies are lightly browned on bottom, 15-18 minutes. Transfer cookies to wire rack and cool completely. Repeat with remaining dough.

NOTE: To toast oats, spread them out over a baking sheet and bake in middle of 350 degree oven until lightly colored, 5 to 6 minutes. To toast almonds, spread them out over a baking sheet and bake in middle of 350 degree oven until fragrant and lightly colored, 8 to 10 minutes.

Vegan Toll House Carob Chip Cookies

As a reformed chocoholic I came up with this recipe one day
when I really needed a fix!!!!! After being unable to find a
vegan toll house cookie, I decided to modify what was out there.
Here is what my family now enjoys.

1 1/4 c. whole wheat pastry flour
1 c. plain, unbleached, all purpose flour
1 t. Featherweight baking powder
1 t. salt
1/3 c. spectrum spread
1/3 c. canola oil
1/3 c. brown sugar
1/3 c. Sucanat
1/3 c. Florida Crystals (evaporated cane juice)
1 t. alcohol free vanilla extract
3 Ener-G egg replacers
6 T. soy milk
2 c. malt sweetened carob chips
1 c. chopped nuts (I use walnuts and pecans)

Sift flour, baking powder and salt into a small bowl. In a large
mixer bowl beat Spectrum spread, oil, sugars, and vanilla until
creamy. Add powdered egg replacer and mix. Slowly beat in
soy milk. Gradually beat in flour mixture. Stir in carob chips
and nuts. Drop by rounded tablespoon onto ungreased baking
sheets.

BAKE in preheated 375 degree oven for 9-11 minutes OR until
golden brown. Cool on baking sheets for two minutes; remove
to wire racks to cool completely.

DOUGH can also be spread into a greased pan. Bake in
preheated oven for 20-25 minutes or until golden brown. Cool
completely in pan on wire rack. Cut into bars.

Peanut Butter Cookies*

3/4-1 c.	honey
2 t.	alcohol free vanilla
3/4 t.	salt
½ t.	alcohol free lemon extract (optional)
1 ½ c.	peanut butter
1/4 c.	oil
1 c.	whole wheat pastry flour
1 c.	oat flour
½ t.	aluminum/baking soda free baking powder-

Featherweight (Optional)

In bowl mix all ingredients together well. Form into small balls and place on cookie sheet. Flatten with fork. Bake at 350 degrees for 12-15 minutes. Watch carefully. Variations: add carob chips.

Yield: 30 small cookies

BEVERAGES/OTHER

Drinking liquids with your meal is not a good idea. Once the digestive process begins, adding cold beverages stops digestion and can lead to indigestion. Water, is the best liquid to drink and is fine to drink all day, **IN-BETWEEN** meals. If you **MUST** drink at all with your meals, a 4-6 ounce serving of fruit juice is all you really need. Try mixing your own favorite fruit juices for a custom blend. Sweet tea, a Southern necessity, is replaced with the recipe below. It is a caffeine free alternative and is sweetened with 100% concentrated fruit juice. Variations of white grape juice or apple juice are excellent choices.

Herbal Iced Tea*

Caffeine-free herb tea of your Choice
(Celestial Seasonings Wild Berry Zinger, Caribbean Kiwi Peach, CranRazz Sunset, and Country Peach Passion are all great choices)
1-12 ounce can 100% White Grape Juice Concentrate

To ½ gallon of water, add 8 tea bags of your choice. Let steep in the refrigerator at least 4 hours. Sweeten to taste with one can concentrated juice.

Medicinal Herb Teas

Peppermint, echinacea, red clover, horehound, chamomile, licorice root, and the like are best used to help the body fight disease. Heat water to boiling, add tea and let steep 10 minutes. Avoid using sweeteners, which can actually reduce tea's effectiveness.

Fruit Punch

1 - 64 oz. bottle apple juice
1 - 48 oz. can pineapple juice
1 - 64 oz. carton orange juice

Mix all ingredients. Chill thoroughly before serving. Serve in punch bowl garnished with orange slices.

Strawberry Daiquiri

We used to like to eat at those restaurants that are named for the day of the week. Since we never drank alcohol, we would order virgin pina coladas and daiquiri. I found this recipe in *Tastefully Vegan*, by Kathryn and Gerard McLane. My son, who loves strawberries, would drink it every day, if I let him.

10 oz. Frozen strawberries
6 oz. Lemonade concentrate
6 oz. Water

Combine ingredients in a blender. Process until well mixed. Add ice cubes until blender is full and blend again until mixture becomes slushy.

Note: If using unsweetened strawberries, add honey, if desired.

Popcorn

Popcorn is a wonderful, healthy food to eat. When you make it, instead of seasoning it with butter and salt, use McKay's Chicken Style Seasoning, nutritional yeast flakes and herbs of your choice.

*These recipes first appeared in the March/April 1998 issue of Message Magazine.

Vegan Vegetarian Meal Ideas for the Month

Whole Grain White Grits Scrambled Tofu* Morning Biscuits* Sliced tomato Red, Purple, Green Grapes	Tossed Salad Baked Potato topped/Black beans, Salsa, Green onions, Tofutti Better Than sour cream Cornbread muffins	Tossed Salad Jamaican Rice/Peas Curried Tofu Callaloo Wheat Bread	Tossed Salad French Dressing* Spinach Quiche/Soy Cheese Veggie Rice* Steamed Yellow Squash	Fruit Salad Banana Muffins	Haystacks Peanut Butter Cookies Auntie Donna's Yum Yum Ice Cream*	Tossed Salad/Dressing Macaroni and Cheez* Baby Green Peas Candied Yams Cornbread*
Whole Wheat Waffles topped/ Tofutti Better Than Sour Cream, Sliced Strawberries Yves Veggie Canadian Bacon	Tossed Salad Homemade Vegetable Soup Cornbread	Tossed Salad Spaghetti/Sauce Cauliflower Garlic Bread	Tossed Salad Stir Fried Vegetables served over Brown Rice	Tossed Salad Oven Roasted Red Potatoes Corn/Lima Succotash Vegetarian Roast Wheat Bread	Vegetarian Sloppy Joes on Whole Wheat Buns Cole Slaw Baked French Fries	Tossed Salad Veggie Lasagne Steamed Broccoli Whole Wheat Garlic Bread
Cooked Oatmeal/raisins, coconut, almonds, dried pineapple Peanut butter toast Sliced orange/grapefruit	Tossed Salad Chili/Soy Cheese Corn Muffin	Tossed Salad Mashed Potatoes Steamed Broccoli Corn on Cob Wheat Bread	Tossed Salad Spanish Rice Vegetarian Enchiladas Fruit Smoothie*	Pita Bread stuffed with Veggie Pasta Salad Shredded Lettuce PA's Pickle Strips Baked Tortilla Chips	Veggie Baked Beans Veggie Hot Dog on Whole Wheat Bun Potato Salad/Soy Mayonnaise	Tossed Salad Yellow Rice Collard Greens* Bean Sausage Cornbread

Pancakes/with pure maple syrup, topped /Shredded Coconut, Chopped Pecans, Vegetarian Sausage Patties, Pineapple Spears	Tossed Salad, Lentil Soup, Soy Cheese Toast, Iced Herb Tea	Vegan Burgers on Whole Wheat Buns/lettuce, tomato, red onion, soy mayonnaise, Macaroni Salad, PA's Pickle Strips	Tossed Salad, Black Eye Peas, Brown Rice, Steamed Cabbage, Baked Sweet Potato, Cornbread	Tossed Salad, Vegetable Pizza/Soy Cheese, Cookies/Ice Cream	Hoagies, Whole Wheat Sub Rolls, Soy Mayonnaise, Soy Cheese, Vegan Deli Slices, Lettuce, Tomato, Red Onion, Black Olives, Oregano, Basil, Olive Oil, Lemon Juice	Tossed Salad, Scalloped Potatoes, Honeyed Carrots*, Steamed Zucchini, Whole Wheat Yeast Rolls
Granola, Soy Milk, Seasonal Fruit Salad, Wheat Toast with Fruit Sweetened Jelly	Tossed Salad, Veggie Pot Pie, Yeast Rolls	Tossed Salad, Noodle Stroganoff, Green Peas, Yeast Rolls				

While we are **used** to eating 3 hearty meals per day, **2 meals with a very light supper**, if at all is really best. Success to you as you begin your new way of life that includes a plant-based, diet.

It really is the **Best Way** to Health!

SUNDAY	MONDAY	TUESDAY	WEDNESDAY	THURSDAY	FRIDAY	SATURDAY

ONE DAY MEAL PLANNER

MEALS	FOOD ITEMS NEEDED	FOODS SERVED
		Whole Grain Bread, Cereal, Pasta, Rice ☐☐☐☐☐☐ __ __ __ __ __ **Vegetables** ☐☐☐ __ __ **Fruits** ☐☐ __ __ **Legume, Nut, Seed, Meat Alternatives** ☐☐ __ **Non-Dairy Milk Products** ☐☐ __ **Other** __ __ __ __

RECIPES/OTHER NOTES

ONE DAY MEAL PLANNER

MEALS	FOOD ITEMS NEEDED	FOODS SERVED
		Whole Grain Bread, Cereal, Pasta, Rice □□□□□□ __ __ __ __ __ **Vegetables** □□□__ __ **Fruits** □□__ __ **Legume, Nut, Seed, Meat Alternatives** □□__ **Non-Dairy Milk Products** □□__ **Other** __ __ __ __

RECIPES/OTHER NOTES

RECIPE MODIFICATION

Getting in the kitchen and experimenting is what makes food taste good to you. If you have some favorite foods that need to be 'vegetarianized', try experimenting with new seasonings and ingredients. Keep record of what you do so that the new food will taste the same every time you do it.

RECIPE

OLD INGREDIENTS	NEW INGREDIENTS
_____	_____
_____	_____
_____	_____
_____	_____
_____	_____
_____	_____
_____	_____
_____	_____
_____	_____

Method

_____

_____

_____

_____

_____

_____

_____

Result

____Do Again   ____Never Do Again

RECIPE MODIFICATION

Getting in the kitchen and experimenting is what makes food taste good to you. If you have some favorite foods that need to be 'vegetarianized', try experimenting with new seasonings and ingredients. Keep record of what you do so that the new food will taste the same every time you do it.

RECIPE

OLD INGREDIENTS   NEW INGREDIENTS

_____   _____
_____   _____
_____   _____
_____   _____
_____   _____
_____   _____
_____   _____
_____   _____
_____   _____

Method

_____
_____
_____
_____
_____
_____
_____
_____

Result

____Do Again   ____Never Do Again

RECIPE MODIFICATION

Getting in the kitchen and experimenting is what makes food taste good to you. If you have some favorite foods that need to be 'vegetarianized', try experimenting with new seasonings and ingredients. Keep record of what you do so that the new food will taste the same every time you do it.

RECIPE

OLD INGREDIENTS	NEW INGREDIENTS
_____	_____
_____	_____
_____	_____
_____	_____
_____	_____
_____	_____
_____	_____
_____	_____
_____	_____

Method

_____

_____

_____

_____

_____

_____

_____

_____

Result

____Do Again   ____Never Do Again

SHOPPING LIST

Breads/Cereals

Fruits/Veggies

Meat Alternatives

Non-Dairy Milks

Other

-NOTES-

-NOTES-

HERE ARE SOME GREAT RESOURCES TO HELP YOU START YOUR NEW WAY OF LIFE!!!

The Holy Bible, any version

Cookbooks
Choices, Quick and Healthy Cooking
More Choices for a Healthy Low-Fat You*
Cheryl D. Thomas-Peters, Review and Herald, 1994, 1997

Country Life, Edited by Diane Fleming, Family Health Publications, Country Life Publishing, 1990

Of These Ye May Freely Eat, A Vegetarian Cookbook, JoAnn Ranchor, Family Health Publications, 1990

Tastefully Vegan,* Kathryn McLane and Gerard McLane, Challedon Publishing Co., 1995, 1998

The Best of Silver Hills*, Eileen and Debbie Brewer, Silver Hills Publishing, Lumby, British Columbia, Canada, 1996

The Taming of Tofu
Kerri Bennett Williamson, Pacific Press Publishing Association, 1991

The 7th Day Diet
Chris Rucker and Jan Hoffman, Random House, 1991

Weimar Institute's *NEWSTART, Lifestyle Cookbook*, Thomas Nelson Publishers, 1997

*my personal favorites

Magazines

Message Magazine - a Christian magazine of contemporary issues, Review and Herald Publishers

Vibrant Life - a magazine for healthful living, Review and Herald Publishers

Lifestyle Centers

Lifestyle Principles Inc., 4296-D Memorial Drive, Decatur, GA 404-299-0188 or 404-299-0366
Battle Creek Lifestyle Health Center, Battle Creek, MI 1-888-830-4120
Lifestyle Center of America, Sulfur, OK, 1-800-596-5480
Silver Hills Guest House, Lumby, BC, Canada (604) 547-9433
Uchee Pines Lifestyle Center, Seale, AL (334) 855-4764
Weimar Institute, Weimar, CA 1-800-525-9192
Wildwood Lifestyle Center and Hospital, Wildwood, GA, 1-800-634-9355

Excellent Reading Choices

ENERGIZED - Adult Daily Devotional-Kuzma, Kuzma, Williams, Review and Herald, 1997

Proof Positive, How to Reliably Combat Disease and Achieve Optimal Health through Nutrition and Lifestyle, Neil Nedley, MD, Nedley Publishers, 1998, Ardmore Oklahoma

Plus 15 Plan for Health Enhancement 15 Days to Lower Blood Pressure and Cholesterol, Samuel L. DeShay, MD, and Bernice A. DeShay, RN, MPH, Upward Way Inc., 1990

The Ministry of Healing, Ellen G. White, Pacific Press Publishing, 1905

The Simple Soybean and Your Health, Mark Messina, Ph.D., and
Virginia Messina, M.P.H., RD, Avery Publishers, 1994

Understanding the Body Organs
Compiled by Celeste Lee, TEACH Services, Inc. , 1992
Abundant Life Ministry P.O. Box 913 Chadron, NE 69337

Recipe Index

Dinner

Entrees

Salads/Dressings/Sauces

Soups

To purchase your own or additional copies of

Somethin' to Shout About!!

Call your local ABC Christian Bookstore at 1-800-765-6955

OR

contact the author by writing to

Orion Enterprises
P.O. Box 830393
Stone Mountain, GA 30083-0007

Fax or Voice Messages 770-484-5840
E-mail: orionenterprises@aol.com